P9-BHS-713

# Irritable Bowel Syndrome

## and
## *the MindBodySpirit Connection*

*7 Steps for Living a Healthy Life
with a Functional Bowel Disorder,
Crohn's Disease or Colitis*

**William B. Salt II, M.D.**
**and**
**Neil F. Neimark, M.D.**

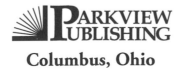

**PARKVIEW
PUBLISHING**

Columbus, Ohio

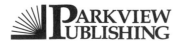
## PARKVIEW PUBLISHING

Parkview Publishing
P.O. Box 09784
Columbus, Ohio 43209-0784

**Credits**
Edited by Joy E. Dickerson
Photography by Susan Salt, except John Lubinsky: 121
Illustrations by Shelley Salt. Also Susan Salt, Annette Aiken and Susan Edison
Front & back cover photography © 1996 Norman Clevenger

**MindBodySpirit Connection Series**
ISBN 0-9657038-5-1
LC 2001098483

**Warning**
This book has been written and published in order to provide people with health information. It cannot serve as a substitute for consultation with a medical doctor. The information in this book is not the same as the practice of medicine and cannot replace or obviate consultation with a physician. The reader can choose, at his/her own risk, to act upon the knowledge and information presented herein. The author and publisher recommend that the reader be aware of his/her health condition and status and consult a physician before beginning any health program, including changes in diet and undertaking an exercise plan.

Publisher's Cataloging-in-Publication Data:

Salt, William Bradley, 1947-
    Irritable bowel syndrome and the mindbodyspirit
connection : 7 steps for living a healthy life with
a functional bowel disorder, Crohn's disease or
colitis / William B. Salt II and Neil F. Neimark. –
Rev. ed.

    p. cm. – (Mindbodyspirit connection series)
    Includes bibliographical references and index.
    ISBN 0-9657038-5-1
1. Irritable colon—Popular works.
I. Neimark, Neil F.  II. Title.
RC862.I77 S35 2002
616.342—dc21

**Printed by Malloy Lithographing, Inc.**
**Ann Arbor, Michigan, U.S.A.**

# Praise

## Early Tributes for
### *Irritable Bowel Syndrome and the MindBodySpirit Connection*

"This is by far the best book on the Mind/Body/Spirit connection that I have read in many years. We have all heard the phrase, 'This book can change your life.' Well, this book really can. It shows you how to use your symptoms as the passport to a better life—physically, emotionally and spiritually."
> – Joan Borysenko, Ph.D.
> Author of *Minding the Body, Mending the Mind* and
> *Inner Peace for Busy People*

"*Irritable Bowel Syndrome and the MindBodySpirit Connection* is must reading for everyone who encounters this common condition—patients, their loved ones, and the health care providers who treat them. Drs. Salt and Neimark have written the definitive healing guide for the millions who suffer from functional bowel problems."
> – Christiane Northrup, M.D.
> Author of *Women's Bodies, Women's Wisdom* and
> *The Wisdom of Menopause*

"A treasury of information to guide your process of healing."
> – Bernie Siegel, M.D.
> Author of *Love, Medicine and Miracles* and *Prescriptions for Living*

"Drs. Salt and Neimark have done a remarkable job in communicating in a clear and concise manner, an understanding of IBS. Through the use of photos and illustrations, and amply referenced, up to date information, the reader can truly begin to acquire the skills to be able to successfully manage this challenging disorder. I will recommend this book to my patients."
> – Douglas A. Drossman, M.D.
> Co-Director, UNC Center for Functional GI and Motility Disorder
> University of North Carolina at Chapel Hill

# Background

## *The MindBodySpirit Connection Series®*

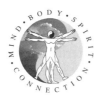 Parkview Publishing offers a new language and way of understanding irritable bowel syndrome and other functional symptoms and syndromes. We consider functional symptoms to be MindBodySpirit Symptoms and functional syndromes to be MindBodySpirit Syndromes. They can both be understood through the interrelationships of mind, body, spirit, environment and society. MindBodySpirit Healing derives from understanding and appreciating the MindBodySpirit Connection, the body's innate healing potential, the individual's responsibility for healing, distinctions between treatment and healing and the power of the patient-doctor relationship. Parkview Publishing is developing a series of books called the MindBodySpirit Connection Series.® *Irritable Bowel Syndrome and the MindBodySpirit Connection* is the first book in the series. The second is *Fibromyalgia and the MindBodySpirit Connection.* Other books on functional symptoms and syndromes are under development.

# Dedication

This book is dedicated to the memory of Dr. Salt's godson, Benjamin Watson Woodruff, born April 27, 1976. Ben was tragically killed in a fire at the Phi Gamma Delta Fraternity house at the University of North Carolina, Chapel Hill, on Mother's Day, May 12, 1996.

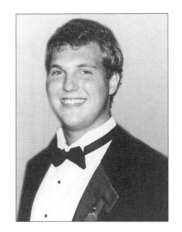

To Ben, his sister Molly and his mother and father Bonnie and Leon:
*We love you. . . . You are never alone.*

### To Ben

I do not remember when we met.
I guess that's because it was before my memory even began.
We've shared so many memories, you and I.
I see us making our drip castles in the sand and
I feel your arm on mine as we lie side by side on a raft.
I taste the salt water we've swallowed so many times.
I hear our laughter as we've grown, and Ben, do I smell our mischief
      (I know our parents do, too).
I can almost see you now, today, looking at me with those beautiful,
      blue eyes, with your hair rumpled.
Only, I can't *touch* you anymore.
You've touched so many lives and you'll never be forgotten.
Because a part of you is with every one of us,
      just as parts of us are with you.
So, you see my friend, you are alive as long as we are.
Though we cannot touch you, we feel you in us
      in our hearts,
      in our thoughts,
      in our actions.
And having had the chance to even know you was a blessing.
Because, you, Ben Woodruff, are an angel.
I love you.

                  – Shelley Salt

# Acknowledgments

We thank Susan Salt, our publisher, artist, photographer, illustrator, communicator and all-around creator. This book, and the MindBodySpirit Connection Series®, exist through her dedication and efforts.

Many friends and colleagues contributed their time and talent. We are particularly indebted to Joy Dickerson, our wordsmith, who used expertise, wit and wisdom to help us massage the manuscript into a much tighter, shorter, polished product than we would have ever thought possible. We give sincere thanks to Mary Ann Hopper, our Quark mastermind, for superior perfectionism, unfailing punctuality and a constant, pleasant "can-do" attitude. We also thank Mary Ann for loyal willingness to help with all of Parkview Publishing's printings, revisions and (now) a new edition, plus layout proficiency with many of our other materials. We are grateful to Shelley Salt, Dr. Salt's daughter, for her wonderful illustrations. We would also like to express appreciation to Michelle Brunetto, Parkview Publishing's office manager and our #1 cheerleader, as well as Gal Friday. Betsy Salt deserves our thanks for the Cataloging in Publication research and exacting guidance on the preparation of the copyright page. Ed Season, as always, we appreciate your insight and vision.

We recognize and thank our photographic models: Joe Brunetto, Michelle Brunetto, Connie Callif, Erin Carruthers, Norman Clevenger, Rose Copp, David Edison, Ruth Harris, Bill Jaeger, Debbie Jaeger, Pat Moloney, Anne Montooth, Casey Salt, Shelley Salt, Chris Season, Mark Thurman, Jenny Walsh, Rick Weber, Bill Wright and Bonnie Woodruff.

We are grateful to our wives and children for their support and patience as we struggled with controlling our own allostatic load while creating this work.

And we thank you, our readers; for without your loyalty and support these words would be in vain.

# Dear Reader

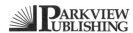

Welcome! Because you've selected our book, we know that you or someone you care about is suffering. We know that you are frustrated and are looking for answers. And we know that you are willing to make a commitment to the exploration of healing.

You've come to the right place! We don't have a simple answer—a pill or potion or quick fix—that will cure irritable bowel syndrome. But, we can offer you a deeper understanding of what causes IBS (and other functional digestive disorders) and how to find significant healing.

The medical field most often treats mind and body as separate. This book not only integrates mind and body, but also adds spirit to your treatment plan. The mind, body and spirit are intimately connected like the ingredients in a loaf of bread. They work together for wellness like flour, water and yeast work together to make a delicious loaf of bread. We will show you how to strengthen these integral ingredients to achieve health and wellness.

Let us help you—as we have helped countless patients—come to peace with your IBS and live a life of greater health, vitality and happiness. We will guide you through The Seven Steps for Living a Healthy Life so that you can move from pain to peace, from helplessness to hopefulness and from frustration to freedom.

Sincerely,

*William B. Salt II MD*

William B. Salt II, M.D.

*Neil F. Neimark M.D.*

Neil F. Neimark, M.D.

# Contents

## Icons Used in This Book

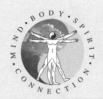

The MindBodySpirit Connection is a term coined by Dr. Salt. It's what makes our books unique and what ties them together. This symbol means that mind, body and spirit are one. Any time you see this icon, be ready for a vital reminder that health is an interweaving of these three components.

This little computer lets you know that you can go to our website for more information on the material being discussed. It's pretty easy; just go to www.parkviewpub.com and click on this icon.

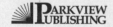

You will really only see this icon in the front and back of the book, but we wanted you to know it's our logo for Parkview Publishing. If you go to our website, you'll see it there, too. It symbolizes a place where you can find friendly, reliable help for your MindBodySpirit symptoms and syndromes.

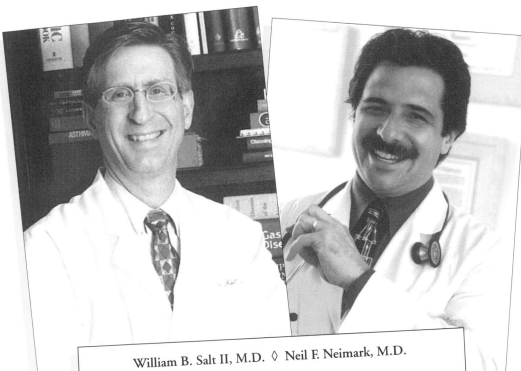

William B. Salt II, M.D. ◊ Neil F. Neimark, M.D.

FOR _**YOU**_
ADDRESS _**120 Elm Street, Anytown, USA**_ DATE _**Today**_

LABEL WITH NAME OF MEDICATION

**R⅄**
- Change your life forever.
- Take control of your IBS or other functional GI disorders.
- Know that your symptoms are distressing and disruptive, but not dangerous.
- Discover the mind-body-spirit connection.
- Use the techniques of mind-body-spirit medicine to help you heal.
- Take the "medicine" from these pages and assume responsibility for your health.
- Use your IBS to turn the negative of illness into the positive of health.
- You have the power to heal and be well.
- You can be healthier than you have ever been before.

_William B. Salt II M.D_        _Neil F. Neimark M.D._

REFILLS
0 • 1 • 2 • 3 • 4 • 5 • 1 YEAR

DEA No. ___**1-888-599-6464**___

# *We Have Your Prescription!*

# Introduction

## *Your Prescription for Change*

> You always had it.
> You always had the power.
> – Glinda, the Good Witch
> in *The Wizard of Oz*

By the time you pick up this book, you have probably spent an untold number of days and nights with recurrent abdominal pain and cramping, unexplained bloating, constipation or diarrhea or all of the above. You may have had multiple visits to your family doctor, gastrointestinal specialist, psychologist or even an alternative healer, all with little or no lasting relief. You may have undergone dozens of blood tests, x-rays, endoscopies, CAT scans and biopsies, all showing that there is nothing wrong. If this sounds like you, do not despair; hope can be found here.

IBS is a major public health topic and receives much attention in newspapers, magazines, radio and television. Many people recognize the acronym *IBS* and terms like *spastic colon, spastic colitis, mucus colitis* and *nervous stomach.* If you suffer from the symptoms of IBS, the most important thing for you to know is that there is hope. Though there is still no cure for IBS, dramatic healing is possible due to new understandings in mind-body-spirit medicine. This new multidisciplinary field of study draws upon the expertise of immunologists, physiologists, research scientists, psychiatrists, psychologists, clergy, neurobiologists, behavioral medicine specialists and others. Due to advances in mind-body-spirit medicine, relief from—and resolution of—many of your symptoms is now within your reach.

# From Frustration to Freedom

IBS is a terribly frustrating disorder! It's frustrating because the symptoms are not only painful and unpleasant, but also because they are embarrassing and often occur at inopportune moments. IBS is frustrating because many doctors don't have helpful advice for sufferers and because written material is often unreliable or is presented as a simple treatment (such as a latest, greatest diet). But with the deeper understanding of IBS that we offer, you will be able to achieve dramatic healing and thereby move from frustration to freedom!

# What Are Functional Gastrointestinal (GI) Disorders?

Functional GI disorders are defined as "variable combinations of chronic or recurrent GI symptoms not explained by structural or biochemical abnormalities." This means that even after performing blood tests, taking x-rays and examining the digestive tract with endoscopy, doctors cannot find a cause for your symptoms.

IBS is the most common functional GI disorder. The symptoms come from the colon and include abdominal pain and bloating, as well as disturbances in defecation (the process of having a bowel movement). These symptoms are diarrhea, constipation and/or alternating constipation and diarrhea. The stool form (bowel movement) is often altered, being lumpy and hard or loose and watery. Other symptoms include straining at having a bowel movement, an urgent need to find a bathroom or a feeling of not having emptied the rectum. Passage of mucus in the stool is also common. The symptoms can be continuous or intermittent.

# You Are Not Alone

Functional GI disorders are common and affect approximately 35 million people in the United States. They account for 10% of visits to primary care doctors and at least 40% of visits to gastroenterologists. IBS affects nearly one out of five people in the United States, from children to the elderly. The average age of onset of IBS is between 20 and 29 years of age. Each year, 2.6 million people seek treatment for symptoms related to functional GI disorders, and visits to physicians total 3.5 million.

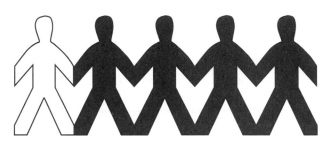

**IBS Affects One in Five Americans**

IBS is a worldwide problem and is prevalent throughout China, the United Kingdom, Australia, New Zealand and Scandinavia. These disorders cost billions of dollars each year in visits to doctors, diagnostic testing and treatments. Furthermore, because IBS is the second leading cause of industrial absenteeism, companies and employers, as well as those who suffer with this disorder, are concerned.

# IBS: The Consequences

Some of the consequences for many who suffer with IBS are:

- Reduced sense of health and well-being
- Constant concerns related to the cause and control of the symptoms
- Sense of a loss of control
- Problems with activities of daily living
- Problems with relationships with family, friends and co-workers
- Disability with missed work days

IBS and other functional GI disorders cause symptoms and discomfort ranging from mild and inconvenient to severe and incapacitating. Current evidence shows that many people with IBS lead restricted lives in multiple areas: diet, social activities, energy level and sense of well-being. Unfortunately, traditional medical science has not been able to offer them much relief.

# "Irritable Body" and Somatization

Just as the GI tract is unusually sensitive and irritable in patients with IBS, many patients with functional GI disorders also seem to have a sensitive or "irritable body." This may lead you to experience many of the constellations of bodily symptoms shown in Table 1. As in IBS, most of the time these "irritable body" symptoms cannot be explained by physical examination, blood tests, x-rays, endoscopic examinations or biopsy results. When this happens, we refer to these medically unexplained symptoms as "functional," "psychosomatic" or "somatization." Most often, disturbances in the mind-body-spirit connection account for much of the trouble.

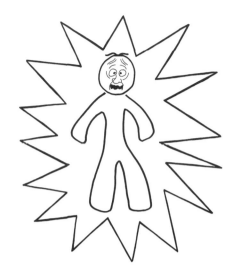

| Table 1 | |
|---|---|
| **Bodily Symptoms: The "Irritable Body"** | |
| Fatigue and low energy | Insomnia and difficulty sleeping |
| Headache | TMJ pain (pain in the jaw) |
| Dizziness | Feeling faint |
| Chest pain | Shortness of breath |
| Back pain | Abdominal pain |
| Painful menstrual periods | Pelvic pain |
| Bladder problems | Decreased sex drive |
| Difficulty thinking and concentrating | |

## Symptoms and Syndromes: "All in Your Head?"

Unfortunately, terms like "functional," "psychosomatic" and "somatization" are often misconstrued to mean that the symptoms are "all in your head," phony or imagined. The truth is that the symptoms are very real. In fact, virtually everyone experiences one or more functional symptoms from time to time. Even mind-body medicine researcher and writer Robert Sapolsky reports intermittent disruptive symptoms. He says, "Personally, all the major rites of passage in my life have been marked by pretty impressive cases of the runs a few days before—my bar mitzvah, going away to college, my doctoral defense, proposing marriage, my wedding, the day my wife gave birth to our son."

However, some people have symptoms that are frequent, constant and severe, and which cause them to consult with doctors. Their symptoms begin to affect every area of their lives. The suffering is enormous. What is going on here? What is the common denominator?

The answer is that the problem is not "all in your head," but is related to the connection between your mind, body and spirit. The mind, body and spirit act together as a system. A disturbance in one causes disturbances in the other two. They contribute together to your level of wellness. You can think of them as a mobile hanging in delicate balance. When you touch or disturb one arm of a mobile, changes are set in motion that affect every other arm of the mobile. Eventually, you hope, the mobile regains its balance. But, sometimes, in the mind-body-spirit relationship, the disturbance is too much. The mind-body-spirit mobile cannot regain its balance. When that happens, illness occurs. And for some people, that illness is diagnosed as irritable bowel syndrome.

## The Mind-Body-Spirit Connection

You will learn in this book that the mind, body and spirit are one. It no longer makes sense to classify problems as either stress/emotional (mind) or physical (body). For example, a physical symptom such as abdominal cramping may trigger or be triggered by emotional stress. The symptom is the same and still needs treatment. You can see that if you treat only mind or only body you will miss out on opportunities for healing. Furthermore, you will discover why it is essential that the mind-body connection include spirit. Scientific evidence continues to confirm the power of spirit and how affirming beliefs—particularly belief in a higher purpose and a higher power—can contribute significantly to your health. A well-nourished spirit is a great preventive measure for many illnesses.

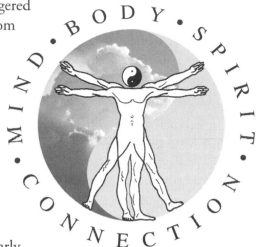

Mind, body, spirit—each is expressed neurochemically in your body. In this book, you will learn about the neurochemical basis of the mind-body-spirit connection. You will find out how to tap into the innate healing potential of your body and the powerful healing forces of your mind and spirit. Most importantly, you will begin to understand that optimal physical health is only possible in the larger context of your emotional, mental and spiritual health. This is the mind-body-spirit connection. With it, you will discover new ways to achieve relief, growth and healing from your IBS.

# Colitis and Inflammatory Bowel Disease (IBD)

The term colitis refers to colon inflammation. It should not be used to refer to IBS because in IBS the colon is not actually inflamed. In IBS, inflammation and other abnormalities in the digestive tract are not present—or at least do not show up on medical tests. However, inflammation is found in several important disorders called inflammatory bowel diseases (IBD). The two types of IBD are ulcerative colitis, which affects the rectum and colon, and Crohn's disease, which can involve both the colon and the small intestine. Nearly one million Americans suffer from IBD.

Although the treatments for irritable bowel syndrome and inflammatory bowel diseases differ, many people with IBD can benefit from the recommendations made in this book. Emotional distress and the stress response can activate or aggravate both IBS and IBD. Furthermore, many people with IBD also have IBS, and recognition of this overlap is important in order to avoid unnecessary IBD treatment. The application of IBS management strategies can be helpful in the management of IBD. Inflammation may be quieted, and symptoms may be relieved.

## Why a Book about IBS?

New developments in the diagnosis and treatment of IBS and new approaches involving the mind-body-spirit connection have opened up new opportunities for healing. As a board-certified gastro-enterologist and a board-certified family practitioner, with more than 45 combined years of experience caring for people with IBS and other functional GI disorders, we will provide you with the information you need.

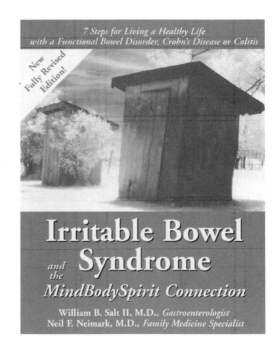

In addition, new restrictions in "managed care" are making it harder for your doctor to spend time with you. In fact, most doctor visits are now limited to 12 minutes or less! Also, managed care makes it more difficult to gain access to medical specialists because your primary care physician is expected to handle most problems and because some specialists are in short supply.

Due to these changes in medicine, you must assume more responsibility for the management of your health care. You will need accurate

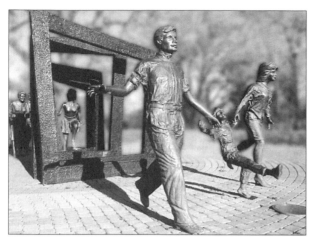

**Step-by-Step to Recovery**

and reliable information. With *Irritable Bowel Syndrome and the MindBodySpirit Connection,* sufferers are finally offered a step-by-step program that leads to a road of recovery.

# You Can Heal!

You are stronger than you think and have more control over your body than you ever realized. The goal of this book is to help you recognize and use the various tools available to tap into your body's powerful ability to heal. Not only can you heal from IBS, but you can turn the negative of your illness into the positive of health and wellness. You can use your diagnosis of IBS to activate the mind-body-spirit connection and become healthier than ever before. The seven steps that you will take are listed in Table 2.

| Table 2 |
| --- |
| ### 7 Steps for Living a Healthy Life with IBS |
| 1. Connecting Your Mind, Body and Spirit<br>2. Understanding the Neurobiology of the MindBodySpirit Connection<br>3. Focusing on IBS<br>4. Choosing to Heal<br>5. Caring for Your Body<br>6. Caring for Your Mind and Spirit<br>7. Taking Action If Symptoms Persist |

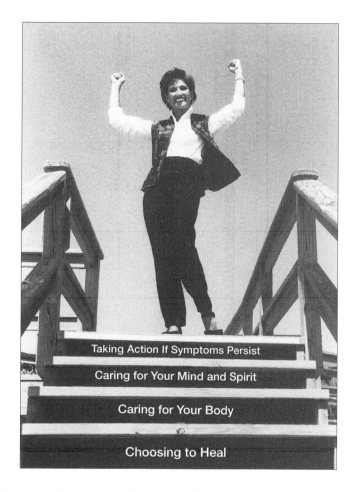

Taking Action If Symptoms Persist

Caring for Your Mind and Spirit

Caring for Your Body

Choosing to Heal

*Focus on the power of your mind rather than on the pain of your digestive symptoms. Use the diagnosis of IBS to realize your ability to heal through mind-body-spirit medicine and become healthier than ever before.*

*Welcome to wellness!*

William B. Salt II, M.D.
Gastroenterologist

Neil F. Neimark, M.D.
Family Practice Specialist

# STEP 1

## CONNECTING YOUR MIND, BODY AND SPIRIT

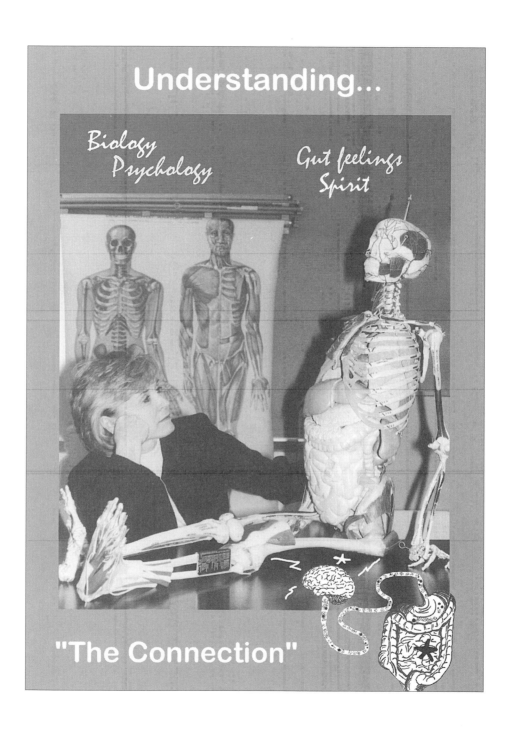

# Chapter 1

## *Symptoms of Distress*

. . . the first stage of healing always begins with breakdown.
The first stage of healing is characterized by a focus on, and
attention to, the external manifestations of distress (symptoms).
– *Intentional Healing*
Elliott Dacher, M.D.


**You are never alone.**
– *The Legend of Bagger Vance*
Steven Pressfield


There is an epidemic of unexplained digestive and abdominal
symptoms—including abdominal pain and discomfort, diarrhea,
constipation and bloating—as well as of other symptoms such as
widespread pain, fatigue and sleeping problems—and practically
everyone experiences them. Doctors call recurrent and bothersome
medically unexplained symptoms "functional."


## Symptoms: Here Today, Gone Tomorrow

At one time or another, almost all of us experience bouts of abdominal
pain and discomfort that can last from minutes to hours to days, but
eventually, our symptoms go away. Sometimes the symptoms arise sud-
denly, such as the vomiting and diarrhea that may occur with food poi-
soning. Sometimes the symptoms are part of a stomach flu or intestinal
infection. Other times, symptoms seem to occur during times of deep
personal difficulty.

A recent study by Dr. Robert Sandler and others from the University of North Carolina confirmed the common occurrence of such gastro-intestinal symptoms when it showed that, in any given month, about 40% of people report one or more digestive symptoms, including abdominal pain, bloating and diarrhea (*Digestive Diseases and Sciences,* June, 2000;45:1166–71). Most people rated these symptoms as moderate to severe in intensity and reported that these symptoms caused some limitation in their daily activities.

In addition to intestinal symptoms, other common symptoms that come and go quite frequently include headache, fatigue, insomnia, body aches and various pains. These symptoms occur so universally that most people usually pay them no mind. Most of these symptoms tend to appear and disappear quite randomly and are generally not associated with any serious underlying medical problem. The benign nature of such symptoms is attested to in the colloquial advice of physicians, "Take two aspirin and call me in the morning." In fact, Dr. Lewis Thomas, in his book *The Lives of a Cell,* states, "The great secret, known to internists and learned early in the marriage by internists' wives, but still hidden from the general public, is the fact that most things get better by themselves. Most things, in fact, are better by morning."

# Functional Symptoms: Here Today, Here Tomorrow

If you are reading this book, you probably have symptoms that are not "better by morning" or that recur so frequently that you are almost always "not well." This constellation of recurring symptoms begins to dominate your life. You find yourself rearranging your schedule to accommodate your pain. You stop making social plans in order to avoid the embarrassment of running to the bathroom all the time. You start to feel isolated, frustrated and overwhelmed, and, one day, you come to believe that you are no longer in control of your life. Your symptoms are in charge.

Eventually, your pain and your sense of isolation lead you to the doctor's office, where your physician—after listening to your symptoms and

Table 1.1

## Functional Gastrointestinal Symptoms*

| | |
|---|---|
| Lump in the throat | Chest pain |
| Swallowing trouble | Heartburn |
| Indigestion | Dyspepsia |
| Upper abdominal pain | Nausea |
| Vomiting | Chronic abdominal pain |
| Attacks of abdominal pain | Abdominal bloating/distention |
| Gas | Belching |
| Flatulence | Chronic/recurrent diarrhea |
| Chronic constipation | Anal or rectal pain |

*Affect two of every three people in the United States.

Research has confirmed that everyone experiences a variety of other functional symptoms from time to time, including those listed in Table 1.2. As with functional gastrointestinal symptoms, there is considerable variability in how long symptoms last, how severe they are and which symptoms are present. 🖳 Learn more about <u>functional symptoms</u>.

# Symptoms That Trouble Can Transform

One of the basic teachings of mind-body-spirit medicine is that optimal physical health is achievable only in the larger context of your mental, emotional and spiritual health. This means that a powerful and sacred *relationship* exists between your body and your mental, emotional and spiritual well-being.

As in any relationship, things may not turn out the way you hoped they would. Divorce is not an option in this relationship. For better or for worse, you are married to your body. It is the only one you get. You do have options, however. You can:

Table 1.2

# Functional Symptoms*

### Body

| | |
|---|---|
| Digestive symptoms (Table 1.1) | Widespread aching and pain |
| Localized bodily pain | Fatigue and low energy |
| Headaches | Temporomandibular joint/jaw pain |
| Dizziness and feeling faint | Shortness of breath |
| Tremulousness and jitteriness | Heart racing or rhythm problems |
| Chest pain | Pelvic pain |
| Back pain | Bladder problems |
| Menstrual symptoms | Sweating |
| Sexual difficulties | |

### Mind

| | |
|---|---|
| Nervousness | Anxiety and panic or phobias |
| Irritability and negative thinking | Obsessions |
| Difficulty thinking/remembering | Depression |

### Spirit

| | |
|---|---|
| Hopelessness | Low self-esteem |
| Feelings of worthlessness | Unhealthy shame |
| Lack of meaning or purpose | Sense of isolation or separation |

*Affect virtually everyone from time to time with variable duration, severity and combinations.

1. kick, scream, fight and stay angry with your body;
2. live in quiet desperation with your body, avoiding and ignoring it; or
3. learn how to care for your body in a way that allows you to find meaning, joy and growth in life, despite your physical limitations.

If you are like most people, you will probably cycle through all of these options from time to time, but the goal of mind-body-spirit medicine is to help you exercise option number three. Yes, you may at times be distressed by your symptoms, frustrated with your body and angry at life and even at God for the physical pain and discomfort you sometimes endure. However, for option number three to become a reality in your life, you must ultimately come to an acceptance of the way things are.

Fritz Perls, the renowned Gestalt therapist, used to say, "Nothing changes until it becomes what it is." In order for you to change your health and your relationship with your body for the better, you must accept it as it is. Right now, you suffer from physical symptoms and the emotional fallout from them is frustrating and depleting. However, in acknowledging your distress, you begin to accept your body for what it is. Then, and only then, can you move beyond your distress into intentional healing. You will learn how to do this in the upcoming chapters. We promise.

Acceptance leads not to surrender but to serenity; not to fear but to freedom. This freedom is the ability to live a full and meaningful life in spite of the limitations of your body. This freedom comes from your soul—the "spirit" component of the mind-body-spirit connection. While your body teaches you that you have limitations, your soul teaches you that the possibilities for love, joy and meaning are limitless.

## Accepting Your Limitations

You don't have to like your limitations in life, but—for healing to occur—you do have to accept them. You can—and should—continue to try to find solutions for your pain and discomfort. But eventually, you must come to understand your physical struggles in the context of your mental, emotional and spiritual health.

What does this mean? It means that you begin to use your body as a teacher to transform you rather than torment you. For example, if your emotional goal is to achieve a sense of inner peace and balance in your life, then when you experience uncomfortable spasms or pain, you can say to yourself, "Okay. I hate this pain. I'm tired of these spasms, but I want to have emotional peace and balance in my life. Therefore, I'm going to let this pain remind me to be patient with my body and my limitations in this very moment of my life. I'm going to learn 'letting go,' inner strength and tolerance." When you begin to view your symptoms in this context, you can take any symptom or pain you experience and ask yourself, "How can this pain teach me to be more loving and more accepting of myself and others?" This simple exercise may ignite in you a deeper compassion for the pain of others. In this way, your very pain leads you beyond yourself into a state of greater love for others: a spiritually powerful place for healing.

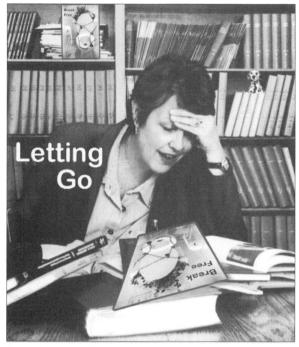

Learning Inner Strength

## Acceptance Is Not Resignation

Don't confuse acceptance with resignation. Acceptance encourages you to make peace with your limitations at the same time that it encourages you to seek out new treatment options to help you reduce your pain. Resignation depletes and depresses you and prevents you from making true peace with your limitations. It may prevent you from even seeking help. Acceptance leads to hope. Resignation leads to hopelessness. Your challenge is to find—and change—the meaning in your pain, even as you seek ways to eliminate and reduce it.

In Chapter 2, you will learn how *people* with functional symptoms become *patients* with functional syndromes.

# Chapter 2

## *Symptoms to Syndromes*

It is being increasingly recognized that a significant amount
of human suffering, medical costs and general loss of
productivity can be attributed to what traditionally have
been labeled "functional" medical disorders or syndromes.
– Emeran A. Mayer, M.D., Gastroenterologist
Director, UCLA/CURE Neuroenteric Disease Program

The term "functional" tends to carry a negative connotation, implying that somehow the symptoms are phoney, imagined or all in your
head. This misconception only leads to frustration and confusion.
New understandings about functional symptoms and syndromes
provide powerful evidence that the mind, body and spirit are in-
extricably linked and, in fact, are one integrated system of health.
The good news is that you can use these new understandings about
the mind-body-spirit connection to get well again.

## *People* with Functional *Symptoms* Become *Patients* with Functional *Syndromes*

Many people with the symptoms described in the first chapter decide to
see a doctor, especially if their symptoms include severe pain, raise concerns about a serious disease like cancer, interfere with life activities (including work, social life and personal relationships) or become associated
with anxiety or depression. Troubling thoughts about these symptoms can
remain constantly in your mind, sapping your energy, interfering with
sleep and causing chronic anxiety, depression, fatigue and inner discord.

"Surely doctors should be able to find out what is wrong with me, make
a diagnosis and prescribe effective treatment," you contend. "After all, look

at all the amazing advances in medicine and surgery today. A cure for me must be just around the corner—a new medication or something. Right?"

Medical research has confirmed that most health care visits are made for common symptoms for which no specific cause can be found. Kurt Kroenke, M.D., from Indiana University, is a world authority on medically unexplained symptoms and syndromes. In a landmark study, Dr. Kroenke found that only 16% of symptoms for which patients consulted with a primary care physician could be medically explained (*American Journal of Medicine,* 1989;86:262–6).

When *people* with functional *symptoms* come to the doctor for help, they often become *patients* diagnosed with functional *syndromes*. A syndrome is a cluster of related symptoms and signs that help a doctor to recognize, diagnose, treat and manage a patient's presenting complaints. Because many of the same symptoms occur in different syndromes, which particular syndrome the patient gets diagnosed with depends upon the predominant symptoms and the type of specialist seen (Table 2.1). Many patients see more than one specialist and receive more than one diagnosis.

Doctors Wayne Katon, Mark Sullivan and Ed Walker, from the University of Washington Medical School, stress that functional medical syndromes that have no clearly defined cause are responsible for a high percentage of visits to specialists (*Annals of Internal Medicine,* 2001;134:917–925). Learn more about <u>functional syndromes</u>.

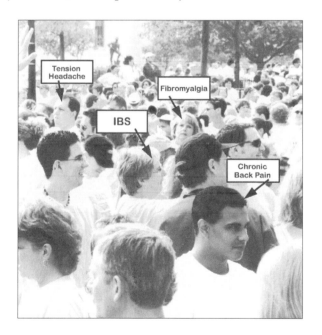

# Functional Gastrointestinal Syndromes

Gastroenterologists have classified 21 functional GI disorders, or syndromes. Patients with functional GI syndromes make up 12% of all

Table 2.1

## The Most Common Functional Syndromes

| Specialist | Diagnosis or Syndrome |
| --- | --- |
| Gastroenterologist | Irritable bowel syndrome (IBS) and/or one or more of 21 functional gastrointestinal disorders |
| Rheumatologist | Fibromyalgia |
| Internal Medicine | Chronic (postviral) fatigue |
| Sleep Specialist | Sleep disorder |
| Psychiatrist or Primary Care Doctor | Depression; Generalized anxiety disorder; Panic disorder; Somatoform disorder |
| Neurologist | Dizziness; Headache |
| Endocrinologist | Hypoglycemia |
| Otolaryngologist (ENT Specialist) | Dizziness; Globus; Tinnitus (ringing in the ears) |
| Dentist | Temporomandibular joint (TMJ) syndrome |
| Cardiologist | Atypical chest pain; Mitral valve prolapse; Palpitations |
| Allergist or Occupational Medicine | Multiple chemical sensitivity |
| Orthopedic Surgeon | Low back pain, Neck pain |
| Urologist | Interstitial cystitis |
| Pulmonologist | Hyperventilation; Dyspnea (shortness of breath) |
| Gynecologist | Pelvic pain; Premenstrual tension Syndrome (PMS); Premenstrual dysphoric disorder (PMDD) |

patients seen by primary care doctors and 40% of all patients seen by gastroenterologists. The three most common functional syndromes seen in gastroenterology are irritable bowel syndrome (IBS), functional dyspepsia (upper abdominal pain and discomfort) and functional chest pain. You will learn about IBS and functional GI symptoms and syndromes in Step 3. Learn more about <u>functional gastrointestinal syndromes</u>.

## Misconceptions, Frustration and Confusion

The diagnosis of functional syndromes is intended to reassure patients that the doctor understands their symptom experience and that there is no serious disease present. Unfortunately, many patients do not understand what is happening to them. How can they feel so ill when all of their medical tests are normal?

Many doctors also have difficulty understanding functional symptoms and explaining them to patients. Functional symptoms and syndromes are often considered to be related to stress, depression, anxiety or psychosomatic reactions. The term "functional" tends to carry a negative connotation, implying that somehow the symptoms are phoney, imagined or all in your head. These misconceptions only lead to greater frustration and confusion.

## Functional Symptoms, Syndromes and the Mind-Body-Spirit Connection

Functional symptoms and functional syndromes are all related to one another. In a recent medical report entitled, *Functional somatic syndromes: One or many?* British physicians Wessely, Nimnuan and Sharpe have reviewed previous studies and conclude that a substantial overlap exists between the individual syndromes and that the similarities between them outweigh the differences (*Lancet,* 1999;354:936–939). We agree and will show you that functional syndromes, including IBS, result from disturbances of the mind-body-spirit connection and its interrelationships with heredity (genetics) and the environment, both physical and social.

You will begin your journey of discovering why you are ill and what you can do to help yourself heal by reading the next chapter on mind, brain and consciousness.

# Chapter 3
## *Mind, Brain and Consciousness*

The bond between mind and the brain is a deep mystery.
— *The Mysterious Flame: Conscious*
*Minds In a Material World*
Colin McGinn

Thus, it is possible for emotions to be triggered in us without
the cortex (mind/brain) knowing exactly what is going on.
— Joseph LeDoux, Ph.D.
Neuroscientist at New York University's Center for Neural Science
and author of *The Emotional Brain*

Brain and mind are not the same. Your brain is part of the visible, tangible world of the body. Your mind is part of the invisible, transcendent world of thought, feeling, attitude, belief and imagination. The brain is the physical organ most associated with mind and consciousness, but the mind is not confined to the brain. The intelligence of your mind permeates every cell of your body, not just brain cells. Your mind has tremendous power over all bodily systems.

## The Relationship of Brain and Mind

The human brain is a three-pound, cantaloupe-sized organ whose external surface has many folded and convoluted contours. These folds and convolutions increase the surface area of the brain, vastly increasing the number of possible connections between brain cells, and thereby increasing the computing power of the brain. Examined under a microscope, each of the brain's 100 billion cells makes approximately 1000 connections—called synapses—with other brain cells. These synapses weave an intricate tapestry of living brain cell fibers, creating the rich and complex communications network called the brain.

The brain is the central processing unit of the body and plays a key role in translating the content of the mind (your thoughts, feelings, attitudes, beliefs, memories and imagination) into complex patterns of nerve cell firing and chemical release. These complex patterns of nerve cell firing and chemical release are called neurosignatures, and they intimately effect the physiology and biochemistry of the body.

# All Life Events Have Neurosignatures

In *Timeless Healing,* Herbert Benson, M.D., states that every event in life is associated with unique and distinct neurosignatures. For example, when you visit a flower garden, visual, auditory and kinesthetic impulses travel from your eyes, ears and sense receptors to your brain, where these sensations are blended with your state of mind (your thoughts, feelings and memories). These signals then trigger a unique and distinct pattern of nerve cell firing and chemical release—a unique neurosignature.

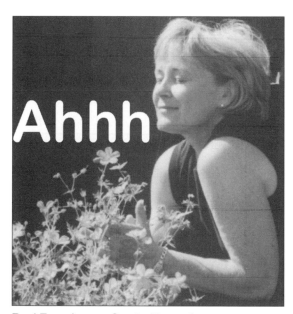

**Real Experiences Create Neurosignatures**

In the case of a calm and peaceful event—like this beautiful garden—the nerve cell firing and chemical release lead to the production and release of calming chemical messenger molecules (which will be discussed further in Chapter 7), which induce a state of bodily calm. Neurosignatures are stored in your mind as memories. Every memory carries with it not only the images, sounds, smells, tastes and touch of an event, but also the thoughts and feelings that were associated with that event.

# Many Kinds of Memory

Memory can occur in many different places, like pictures stored in different photo albums. The four places where memory is stored are:

1. **Your body.** Memories stored here are called body memory, muscle memory or cellular memory.
2. **Your unconscious mind.** These are memories of events, feelings, images or situations of which you have no conscious memory. They remain stored in your mind like a misplaced photo album.
3. **Your conscious mind.** These are memories of events, feelings, images or situations of which you are consciously aware.
4. **Your soul.** Many religious traditions believe that the soul carries memories of your sacred connection with a divine presence or God, and in this sense, a large part of spiritual healing is remembering. That is why spiritual growth often comes intuitively through remembering sacred connections. Some also feel soul memory is present in terms of a conscience that knows what is right and wrong.

## Body memory

An important component of the mind-body-spirit connection is realizing that your body can remember things without your mind being conscious of them. This is called body memory. Every musician knows about body memory. It is what allows you to play a piece of music without having to think about every note and rhythmic change. After sufficient practice, your fingers seem to play the piece of music on their own. Do you remember learning how to drive a stick shift? Do you remember how much conscious effort it initially required to shift smoothly? Now your body does it unconsciously, at the level of body memory. These are forms of body memory.

Let's look now at how the body, through the mechanism of visualization, can create memories of things that haven't even occurred yet.

# Visualizations Create Neurosignatures

We already discussed how the sensory input from an external event, like a flower garden, enters the brain and blends with the mind to create a neurosignature (distinct pattern of nerve cell firing and chemical release). This particular kind of neurosignature creation is called "bottom-up" because it moves from the outside of your body up to your brain.

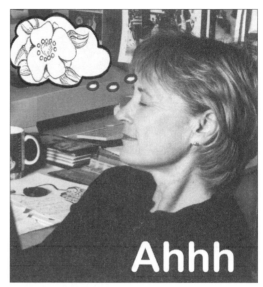

**Remembered Experiences Create Neurosignatures**

There is a second way to create neurosignatures: by evoking an image or recalling an event in your mind and imagination. When you imagine strolling in a beautiful garden on a warm and sunny day and enjoying the delicious fragrances, a new neurosignature is created. If this memory is of an actual garden that you've walked in before, it triggers the original neurosignature you first felt when walking in that very garden. When you create a neurosignature from your imagination or by evoking a memory of an actual event, this is called "top-down," because the neurosignature evolves from the top (brain) and moves down into your body through the release of chemical messenger molecules and patterns of nerve cell firing.

## The difference between a real event and a vividly imagined one

Recent scientific data support the intriguing fact that your body cannot tell the difference between a real event and one that you vividly imagine. This amazing mind-body connection makes sense when you understand neurosignatures. Whether the neurosignature is evoked top-down or bottom-up, the pattern of nerve cell firing and chemical release is similar.

Kosslyn and Albert performed PET (Positron Emission Topography) studies where they viewed the areas of the brain that "lit up" when patients experienced certain events or recalled them from memory. The PET scan technology showed that the same parts of the brain were activated whether people actually experienced something or just vividly imagined it (*Journal of Cognitive Neuroscience,* 5;1993;263–87). This research shows how powerful neurosignatures are in allowing your mind to influence your body, as well as the power of your body to influence your mind. As Norman Cousins says, ". . . the human mind converts ideas and expectations into biochemical realities."

You might better understand the power of visualization to create memories of things that haven't yet happened when you think of a flight simulator. By anticipating events before they happen, pilots can create body memories for how to handle situations when they really do occur. In this sense, neurosignatures (created through the imagination) translate the invisible elements of mind (thought, feeling, attitude, belief and imagination) into visible forces of biochemistry that communicate your thoughts and feelings to the cells and organs of your body. You are conscious of some of these communications; others are unconscious.

## Your Conscious and Unconscious Mind

Webster's dictionary defines consciousness as "awareness, especially of something within oneself." In this sense, your conscious mind refers to your awareness of your own thoughts, images, feelings, attitudes, beliefs and sensations. Raising your consciousness implies raising your awareness of your own thoughts, feelings and bodily sensations. This awareness is critical to all forms of healing.

The unconscious mind represents that part of your life experience of which you are unaware. When it comes to your health and healing, the unconscious dimension of your mind is as important as your conscious mind. The unconscious mind is likened to the part of an iceberg that remains underwater. Your conscious mind, likened to the tip of the iceberg, represents only a small fraction of your total mind (conscious plus unconscious).

Neuroscience confirms that much of what we experience as symptoms of the mind and body are related to processes and responses within us that occur at an unconscious level. In fact, neuroscientist Candace Pert believes that part of the unconscious mind may actually be in the body, at the level of cellular memory.

# The Malleable Brain

The brain is not a rigid structure. In fact, the brain is extremely malleable, continually reorganizing itself and changing its structure and synaptic connections. Scientists refer to the brain's inherent capacity for change as "plasticity." In this sense, the brain is like Play-doh in its capacity for molding, change and healing. Paula Tallal, co-director of the Center for Molecular Neuroscience at Rutgers University in Newark, NJ (Sharon Begley, *Newsweek,* January 1, 2000) says, "You can create your brain from the input you get."

In *The Art of Happiness,* the Dalai Lama and Howard C. Cutler, M.D., suggest that brain plasticity "appears to be the physiological basis for the possibility of transforming our minds. By mobilizing our thoughts and practicing new ways of thinking, we can reshape our nerve cells and change the way our brains work." This remarkable feature of the brain allows you—through conscious awareness, concentration and repetitive practice—to rewire and remold your neural connections, creating new neurosignatures for health, happiness and peace of mind.

# What You Don't Know Can Hurt You

As you consider the attributes of the conscious and unconscious mind, you begin to see that all healing represents a movement from the invisible to the visible, from unconsciousness (unawareness) to consciousness (awareness). Mind-body-spirit medicine teaches you how to connect the invisible world of mind (thought, feeling, attitude, belief and imagination) and spirit (soulfulness, a sense of meaning and purpose, connection to a higher power) with body (the visible world of physical health and well-being). Understanding this connection is vital because, when it comes to health and healing, what you don't know (what is invisible to you) can hurt you. Bringing unconscious feelings into conscious awareness may be painful, but it allows healing to begin. In the light of conscious awareness, you can process your feelings in a way that heals rather than harms.

Understanding the mind-body-spirit connection provides you with powerful tools for processing the inevitable array of troubling thoughts, feelings and spiritual crises that accompany any serious or chronic illness. Though the task of conscious growth seems daunting, always remember that you have more power and control over your mind, body and spirit than you may be aware of. In fact, the awareness of what you are unaware of—exactly how much power you have—changes you and gives you greater power to heal.

In the next chapter, we'll introduce the mind-body connection.

# Chapter 4
## *Mind and Body*

*. . . investigators discovered what shamans have long known, that the mind and the body are one.*
— *Shaman, Healer, Sage*
Alberto Villoldo

This is Descartes' error: the abysmal separation between body and mind . . . the suggestion that reasoning, and moral judgment, and the suffering that comes from physical pain or emotional upheaval might exist separately from the body. Specifically: the separation of the most refined operations of the mind from the structure and operation of a biological organism.
— *Descartes' Error*
Antonio R. Damasio, M.D.

---

You know that your mind and body are connected: think about the muscle tension, sweating, rapid heartbeat and shortness of breath that occur in any anxiety-provoking situation.

---

## The Mind-Body Connection

Do you remember?

- The nausea and stomach upset you felt before giving that big speech? Perhaps you are one of a majority of people who experience unpleasant symptoms every time you are called upon to speak in public.

- The cramps and diarrhea you experienced before your big job interview?
- That funny feeling in your stomach when you first fell in love?
- The "butterflies" before the big game?

People differ in their awareness (consciousness) of the connection between mind and body. Some people are exquisitely sensitive to the signals that the mind and body send back and forth to one another, and some are not.

Symptoms that arise from the connection between mind and body are common and normal. Many times, these symptoms are associated with heightened stress or painful feelings. Sometimes the symptoms arise from the mind (troubled thoughts, feelings or memories) and the body pays the price (palpitations, sweating, indigestion). Sometimes the symptoms arise from the body (viral illness or infection) and the mind pays the price (feeling miserable or depressed).

## Mind-Body Medicine

The field of mind-body medicine teaches that the invisible energies of thought, feeling, attitude, belief and imagination are manifested in your physical body, stirring the very fabric of your physiology and biochemistry. These invisible energies can be harnessed to aid in the treatment—and prevention—of disease.

Researchers at Harvard Medical School have been studying the benefits of mind-body interactions for more than 25 years. They have shown that when a person engages in a repetitive prayer, word, sound or phrase while passively disregarding intrusive thoughts, a specific set of physiologic changes ensues. In what Harvard's Dr. Herbert Benson calls the "relaxation response," there is a slowing of metabolism, heart rate, respiratory rate and brain waves.

These changes are brought about by the focused attention of the invisible forces of the mind; yet they create remarkable changes in the visible physiology and biochemistry of the body. Over two decades of research by Dr. Benson and his colleagues at Harvard show that regular elicitation of the relaxation response brings about positive health benefits for numerous conditions, including high blood pressure, irregularities of heart rhythm, many forms of chronic pain, insomnia, infertility, symptoms of cancer and AIDS, premenstrual syndrome, anxiety and mild to moderate depression.

## Physical Abnormalities Versus Symptoms

As you begin to link the mind and body, you will start to see the distinctions between physical disorders and how your mind perceives them. In medical practice, bodily symptoms generally fall into two major categories:

1. Those that can be correlated (through the results of laboratory testing or imaging studies) with visible and identifiable physical or biochemical abnormalities, and
2. Those that cannot be correlated with any visible or identifiable physical or biochemical abnormality.

There can be a remarkable discordance between the perception of pain (experienced in the mind) and any actual physical abnormality (experienced in the body). This is reflected in an axiom of pain management that says, "Pain is in the body, suffering is in the mind." Philosophically, this phrase translates into the modern colloquialism, "Pain is inevitable, suffering is optional."

# IBS: Symptoms Without Physical or Biochemical Abnormalities

You know that the symptoms of IBS are not explained by currently available medical tests like blood tests, x-rays and flexible sigmoidoscopy or colonoscopy. In Steps 2 and 3 of this book, you will see how and why your symptoms occur. New neuroscientific understandings are blurring the distinction between symptoms with and symptoms without identifiable physical or biochemical abnormalities.

But for now, realize that there is nothing phony or imaginary about symptoms that do not correlate with physical or biochemical abnormalities. The abdominal pain and bowel problems of IBS are real.

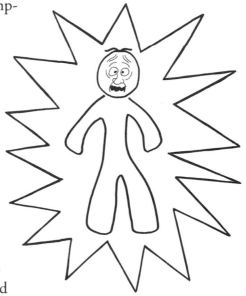

The phenomenon of functional symptoms (those that don't correlate with any visible or identifiable physical or biochemical abnormality) cannot be understood without understanding the mind-body connection. Functional symptoms affect nearly every body system and occur because of alterations or abnormalities in the way that the mind processes pain and sensation. Perceived stress, emotional pain, undue anxiety, troubling thoughts

**Suffering from Medically Unexplained Symptoms**

and cellular memory are integrally related to your IBS. They affect and influence to what extent and degree you experience symptoms, whether you feel ill with them, whether you miss work or social opportunities and whether you will report them to your doctor.

The mind-body connection is critical to understanding not only IBS and other functional syndromes but also all human disease. Understanding this connection is central to self-care, the achievement of health and wellness and intentional healing.

## A Brief History of the Mind-Body Connection

Throughout history, philosophers and thinkers have considered two different views—that the mind and body are part of the same system and that they are entirely separate. In *Timeless Healing,* Harvard's Herbert Benson, M.D., says, "A review of ancient history shows that we are returning to original beliefs that the mind and body cannot be separated."

In her book, *Health Psychology,* Shelley Taylor says that most evidence suggests that ancient people considered the mind and body as a unit and believed that evil spirits caused disease by entering the body. Exorcising and removing these spirits from the body could restore health. Later, the Greeks attributed disease to body factors (the humoral theory of illness) but believed that these factors could also affect the mind. They proposed the concept of "Holos," that medical disease involved the whole person instead of only the diseased body part. This is the view held by many non-Western societies.

During the Middle Ages, the pendulum swung back toward mental explanations for illness. Disease and illness were felt to be God's punishment for evil doing. A cure was often sought by torturing the body to drive out evil spirits. Later, this "treatment" was replaced by penance achieved through prayer and good works.

With the Renaissance came advances in understanding the human body and disease based upon scientific discovery and new technology, particularly the microscope. Medicine turned more and more to scientific investigation of the body—rather than the mind—as the basis for medical progress. In order to break with the superstition of the past, the whole person was dissected into the mind and body.

In 1637, the French philosopher and mathematician René Descartes suggested that the body did not require the mind to operate. Physicians followed his lead for the next 300 years, emphasizing abnormalities at the cellular level as the sole cause of illness. Physical evidence became the only basis for diagnosis and treatment of illness. This became the biomedical model of illness and health.

## The Biomedical Model of Illness and Health

The biomedical model has governed the thinking of most health practitioners for the past 300 years. It holds that all illness can be explained biologically and assumes that psychological and social processes are independent of the disease process. The biomedical model emphasizes a mind-body dualism in which the mind and the body function as separate entities. In this model, the treatment of illness is emphasized over the promotion of health and health is viewed as the absence of disease.

## From the Biomedical to the Biopsychosocial Model

It was not until the early 1900's, with the work of Sigmund Freud and the rise of modern psychiatry, that physical health began to be reintegrated with the psychological and social environment. Freud's original ideas about compulsion neuroses laid the foundation for a more integrated model of health. Basically, Freud's concept of compulsion neuroses states that if you don't work it out (your troubled thoughts, feelings or images) you'll act it out (either through mental illness or physical illness).

Drawing on Freud's concepts and more completely reintegrating the mind and the body, George Engel, M.D., proposed the biopsychosocial model of illness and health in the late 1970's. Engel's biopsychosocial model holds that multiple factors—biological (physical, neurochemical), psychological (thoughts, feelings, attitudes and beliefs) and social (interpersonal relationships)—are interrelated elements of health. For example, the presence or absence of social support, high levels of stress, depression and physical/biochemical abnormalities interact at the cellular level to produce a state of health or illness. The biopsychosocial model of health proposes that health and illness are caused by multiple factors and produce multiple effects. The mind and body are not separate in relation to issues of health and illness because they both influence the state of health.

Dr. Engel trained Douglas A. Drossman, M.D., a gastroenterologist from the University of North Carolina. Dr. Drossman has pioneered the application of the biopsychosocial model to digestive illness and health (see Chapter 39, "Centers of Excellence"). Dr Drossman says, "To have any chance of clinical success, a management strategy for irritable bowel syndrome (IBS) must integrate psychologic, social and biologic factors, all of which influence the pathophysiology and clinical course of the disease process."

IBS and other functional symptoms and syndromes can only be understood by looking through the lens of the biopsychosocial camera at the mind-body connection. As you change your focus from symptoms to the underlying biological, psychological and social causes, you will be able to develop a better picture of your health. You will discover the causes of IBS in Chapter 11.

The biopsychosocial model emphasizes the promotion of health as well as the treatment of illness. The implication of this for you is that achieving health is an *active* process—in which you must participate fully—rather than a *passive* process, in which some drug, pill or treatment will cure you. The biopsychosocial model teaches that the maintenance of health is a dynamic and ever-changing process. You can take an active role in tending to your biological, psychological and social needs.

In his book, *The Healing Mind,* Paul Martin, Ph.D., writes, "I hope I have convinced you of some simple but far-reaching truths. That our mental state and physical health are inexorably intertwined. . . . That the relationship between mind and health is mediated by both our behavior and by biological connections between the brain and the immune system. That these connections work in both directions, so our physical health can influence our mental state. That all illnesses have psychological and emotional consequences as well as causes."

## Another Dimension to the Connection

But there is another dimension to the mind-body connection. University of Toronto gastroenterologist Nicholas Diamant, M.D., says, "Another dimension is also present and not included in available models, has been a part of all human existence as far as we know, and is a common theme within the concepts of traditional healing practices . . . this dimension includes a connectivity that goes beyond the finite to encompass a unity of mind, body and the universal infinity. Health is seen as a harmonization within this broader unity and disease as a loss of this harmony" (*4th International Symposium on Functional Gastrointestinal Disorders,* 2001, Milwaukee, Wisconsin).

Explore this additional dimension in the next chapter.

# Chapter 5

## *Mind, Body and Spirit: The Connection*

*. . .* investigators discovered what shamans have long known, that
the mind and the body are one. But investigators missed one
element that is the crux of all shamanic healing: the Spirit.
– *Shaman, Healer, Sage*
Alberto Villoldo

---

The healing power of faith is not a new idea, but scientific studies
are increasingly documenting the health benefits of spirituality and
religion. Evidence is accumulating that faith, spirituality, belief in a
higher power and prayer are vital pathways for health and healing.
There is a mind-body-spirit connection.

---

## A Faith That Heals

In 1910, Sir William Osler, perhaps the best-known physician and propo-
nent of modern scientific medicine, wrote of "the faith that heals." His
insights into the healing power of faith—almost a century ago—are just
beginning to be demonstrated in modern scientific studies.

In a recent conference (December 2000) on faith and healing, Harold
G. Koenig, M.D., psychiatrist and author of *The Healing Power of Faith*,
summed up the results of hundreds of scientific studies on religious involvement and health. Dr. Koenig defined religious involvement as a combination of:

1.  Strong personal belief and faith and
2.  Involvement with that faith either by:
    a.  private religious activities (prayer and/or scripture reading)
    b.  use of religion to help cope with stress

    c.  attendance at religious services

    d.  participation in congregational activities

Dr. Koenig believes that "religious involvement is a protective factor that can be quantified like other health variables such as diet, exercise, smoking or alcohol use." In a recent summary analysis, Dr. Koenig found the following positive correlations with religious involvement: greater levels of well being, hope and optimism; greater sense of purpose and meaning; less depression and more rapid recovery; decreased risk of suicide; decreased anxiety and fear; greater marital satisfaction and less risk of divorce; greater social support, which confers health benefits; decreased risk of substance abuse; and lower rate of juvenile delinquency.

## What is spirituality?

Although there are many different definitions, the most useful one from the standpoint of mind-body-spirit medicine is that spirituality is a sense of belief in a higher power and a higher purpose. A *higher power* is something greater than yourself, most often defined as God or a Divine Spirit, but sometimes conceptualized as nature, community, love or truth. A *higher purpose* has to do with the idea that life has meaning and value; that there is an order and a purpose to life and creation; and that you play a vital role in helping to make the world a kinder, more loving and more beautiful place. Having a higher purpose includes having higher values, which include a fundamental belief in the sacredness, worth and dignity of each individual.

    The essence of spirituality lies in the individual's ability to reach beyond his or her own self-centered ideas, concerns and desires and connect with something outside of oneself. Spirituality leads to a sense of meaning, belonging and connectedness.

    Spirituality begins with the realization that—as a human being—you have limitations. John Bradshaw, author of *Healing The Shame That Binds You*, says that the very basis of our spirituality is the "permission to be human, to know that we will make mistakes, that we have limitations." Being human means coming to terms with your imperfections and limitations. In so doing, you are reminded that there is something greater than yourself.

## The difference between spirituality and religion

We (Bill and Neil) believe that the goal of all religions is spirituality. Religion includes cultural rituals, rules and practices that vary in great measure from one religion to another, but which are all designed to help you achieve a connection to a divine being (God or a higher power), a higher purpose and sacred values (the inherent worth and dignity of every human being). If you view spirituality—connectedness to God and a higher purpose in life—as the final destination, then the many religions are different roads that lead there. Huston Smith, author of *The World's Religions,* says that, "Religion confronts the individual with the most momentous option life can present. It calls the soul to the highest adventure it can undertake: the call to confront reality and master the self. The enduring religions at their best contain the distilled wisdom of the human race" *(The Wisdom of Faith with Huston Smith: A Bill Moyers Special).*

# Reintegrating Spirit into Mind-Body Medicine

In *Timeless Healing,* Herbert Benson, M.D., says that we are all "wired for God." His analysis of the scientific literature leads him to conclude that spirituality and religious faith enhance almost all forms of healing. He says that *what* we believe is less important than *that* we believe. Benson's groundbreaking discovery of the Relaxation Response (in his book of the same name), has led him to conclude that the human biological mechanism is set up to function most efficiently when faith, hope and belief in a divine being are present. Whether you are Christian, Jewish, Muslim, Hindu, Buddhist or something else, your belief in a higher power heals.

In their recent book, *Why God Won't Go Away: Brain Science and the Biology of Belief,* researchers Andrew Newberg, M.D., Eugene D'Aquili, Ph.D., and Vince Rause used high tech imaging devices to examine the brains of meditating Buddhist monks and Franciscan nuns. Their data showed that the mystical experiences of the subjects "were not the result of some fabrication, or simple wishful thinking, but were associated instead with a series of observable neurological events." In other words, the "mystical experience is biologically, observably and scientifically real . . ."

Based on a wealth of scientific research, experiential reports and preliminary investigational literature, we conclude that spirituality must be reintegrated into the mind-body connection. The healing power of spirituality is an integral and inseparable part of all other forms of healing.

# Mind-Body-Spirit Medicine: The Biopsychosocialspiritual Model of Health

You learned about the biopsychosocial model of health in the last chapter. We propose that the new term "biopsychosocialspiritual" be introduced to reflect medical professional language for the interrelatedness of the mind-body connection with spirituality, heredity and the environment, both physical and social. In short, mind-body-spirit medicine is the biopsychosocialspiritual model of illness and health.

There are those who propose that belief in science contradicts belief in faith and spirituality. However, throughout history, some of the most brilliant and renowned scientists have held a deep awe and appreciation for the mystery of spirit. Albert Einstein said, "Religion without science is blind, but science without religion is lame." Issues of spirituality are now being brought into mainstream medical education, research and patient care. Many medical schools offer courses and conduct research on religion and spirituality in medicine. For example, Duke University's Center for the Study of Religion/Spirituality and Health conducts research that explores the effects of religious/spiritual beliefs and practices on physical and mental health. Their Internet location is http://www.geri.duke.edu/religion/Homepage.HTML. A recent scientific study showed that persons who attended religious services had significantly lower mortality than those who did not attend (*American Journal of Public Health, 88*:1469, 1998).

## Viewing the mind-body-spirit connection

Let's look at a simple example of how the mind-body-spirit connection works in an actual IBS situation. The general concept is that significant pain in the *body* most often causes uncomfortable thoughts and feelings *(mind)* as well as *spirit*ual anguish. Stressful thoughts and feelings (*mind* stress) usually lead to imbalance in your physical *body* as well as *spirit*ual imbalance. When you suffer from *spirit*ual stress or malnutrition, you often suffer from *body* ailments as well as troubling thoughts and feelings *(mind)*. Figure 5.1 shows how it works.

## The Mind-Body-Spirit Connection

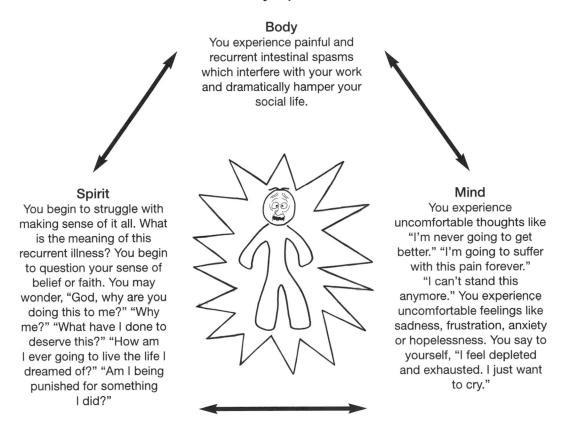

**Body**
You experience painful and recurrent intestinal spasms which interfere with your work and dramatically hamper your social life.

**Spirit**
You begin to struggle with making sense of it all. What is the meaning of this recurrent illness? You begin to question your sense of belief or faith. You may wonder, "God, why are you doing this to me?" "Why me?" "What have I done to deserve this?" "How am I ever going to live the life I dreamed of?" "Am I being punished for something I did?"

**Mind**
You experience uncomfortable thoughts like "I'm never going to get better." "I'm going to suffer with this pain forever." "I can't stand this anymore." You experience uncomfortable feelings like sadness, frustration, anxiety or hopelessness. You say to yourself, "I feel depleted and exhausted. I just want to cry."

**Figure 5.1**

This example reveals that pain in the body can rarely be separated from pain in the mind or pain in the spirit. In general, the stress response in any system (mind, body or spirit) flows in all directions.

# The Bigger Connection

Episcopal Priest Barbara Brown Taylor says that instead of a machine, the universe is most like a web, which shakes and moves and responds to every single stimulus on or in it. "Physical reality," she says, "refuses to be compartmentalized. As hard as we may try to turn it into a machine, it insists on acting like a body, animated by some intelligence that exceeds the speed of light" ("The Luminous Web," *The Christian Century,* June 2–9, 1999).

Your mind, body and spirit are connected to one another in the web of the universe in the same way that you are connected—in some way—to all other human beings in the world. This principle of being connected to all other human beings is part of all great religious traditions that teach that in the oneness of life, is the oneness of the divine.

# Eternity Medicine

Larry Dossey, M.D., is a pioneer in mind-body medicine who provides scientific and medical proof that the spiritual dimension works in healing. Dossey writes that we are entering a new era in medicine, "Eternity Medicine." In his book, *Reinventing Medicine,* he says, "The mind is infinite. This means that my mind touches and is touched by those of everyone else, and that all minds are linked together." Dossey explains that the mind and spirit are eternal and are factors in people helping themselves to heal (through individual prayer) and helping others to heal (through intercessory prayer).

In the next chapter, you will learn more about mind-body-spirit medicine and healing.

# Chapter 6

## *The Language of MindBodySpirit Medicine*

Like the meridians as they approach the poles, science, philosophy, and religion are bound to converge as they draw nearer to the whole.
— *The Phenomenon of Man*
Pierre Teilhard de Chardin

> Unseen energies of thought, feeling, memory, attitude, belief and imagination become manifest in the physical body, stirring the very fabric of our physiology and biochemistry. This understanding reveals why most of the symptoms that cause people to see doctors cannot be explained by conventional medical tests. People, patients and doctors are—and will remain—frustrated until there is a shared appreciation for how the power of these unseen energies affects our physical health. All forms of healing involve making the invisible visible. MindBody-Spirit is a new language of connection, medicine and healing.

## A Failure to Communicate

The last century saw remarkable advances in biomedical technology and treatment. As a society, Americans have come to expect that effective treatments should be available for most medical conditions. Yet, you have already learned that most of the symptoms, syndromes and illnesses that people experience cannot be explained by currently available medical tests. Many patients consult with multiple specialists for functional symptoms and syndromes that no one sees as in any way related.

As a patient, you already know how frustrating it is to have real—and distressing—symptoms, only to be told that all the tests are normal. Even more frustrating is leaving your doctor's office without knowing why you are having these symptoms and what you can do about them.

As doctors, we share your frustration, unable to offer any clear, satisfactory and effective treatment plan. Let's take a look at this problem from the perspective of the patient, the doctor and then the patient-doctor relationship.

## The patient's perspective

When you hear your doctor say that all your tests are normal and that your condition is functional or psychosomatic, you may misunderstand your doctor to be saying that:

- Your symptoms are not real.
- You are just stressed out.
- You must have a mental illness or serious psychological problem.
- There may be a serious disease present that your doctor just can't identify yet.
- Now that there is a diagnosis, taking some pills or a couple of shots should cure you.

Many people and patients do not accept the mind-body-spirit connection because they do not understand it.

## The doctor's perspective

As doctors, we are trained to correctly diagnose medical problems and then identify clear and effective treatment plans to help you feel better. When we are unable to help our patients, we sometimes feel like failures. When we diagnose a patient with IBS, we feel a sense of impotence, frustration and helplessness because we know IBS is a difficult problem to treat and there is no single effective cure.

Because worsening of IBS is very often related to stress, we sometimes wonder if you are just depressed, overstressed, overextended or overanxious. We know that it takes a lot of time—which we don't have—to fully evaluate the psychological and social factors that could be contributing to your IBS, and so we may offer simplistic advice like "just take it easy, relax a little," "maybe you're just too stressed," "maybe you should take some time off work," or "you may have to learn to just live with this." Since we know that your symptoms are not dangerous, we may tend to just dismiss them and say, "Don't worry about it, things could be worse. You'll be okay."

In general, we feel too rushed in a normal office visit to properly evaluate your problem and all the possible treatment options. Also, doctors who don't understand the mind-body-spirit connection believe that IBS is just about stress and may not take your IBS seriously, feeling that it is not a "real" disease. Additionally, doctors are frustrated because managed care has created a situation in which rushed encounters and declining reimbursements prevent us from spending the time necessary to really help you with your problems.

## The Patient-Doctor Relationship

An open, trusting and communicative relationship between patient and doctor is a vital pathway for health and healing. A positive belief and expectancy generated by the relationship between patient and doctor triggers powerful biochemical healing pathways that you will learn about in Steps 3 and 4. Stan Sateren, M.D., of Mt. Carmel Health in Columbus, Ohio, says, "The spirit of dialogue provides opportunities for healing."

Unfortunately—more than ever—there seems to be a failure to communicate and a lack of open dialogue. In his book, *Doctors and Their Patients: A Social History,* Dr. Edward Shorter, professor of medical history at the University of Toronto, writes, "With each passing year, the gap between doctor and patient widens, as doctors retreat increasingly into a shell of resentment and patients become ever more exasperated with the impersonality of care." This widening gap—this failure to communicate—translates into feelings of frustration and unhappiness for both patients and doctors. Furthermore, as we said, many patients and doctors either do not understand or do not accept the mind-body-spirit connection; consequently they underestimate the power of the mind, body and spirit to heal. Only a common language and an openness to dialogue can lead to the convergence of science, religion and philosophy necessary to unleash the healing potential of seemingly diverse healing disciplines.

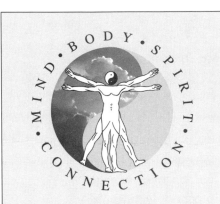

Our logo, seen above, is a combination of different cultural symbols that share similar ideals regarding the MindBodySpirit Connection. The familiar central figure is derived from the Roman architect Vitruvius, which was later studied and utilized by the Renaissance artist Leonardo Da Vinci to illustrate the proportions of the human body. During the Renaissance, there was strong interest both in the body's form as well as in the mind's potential for knowledge. This belief came from the ancient Greek and Roman civilizations where the importance of having a sound/healthy body went hand in hand with having a sound/ healthy mind. Our representation of the figure suggests this balance.

(continued on next page)

# Convergence: Symptoms, Syndromes, Healing Traditions, Science and Language

For thousands of years, people with symptoms and illness from all societies have turned to healers who rely upon the natural capacity of the body to heal through physiologic bodily systems activated by states of mind. Universal concepts and beliefs among prehistoric shamans and healers from Chinese, Aryuvedic (a tradition in India), Native American and Western Hippocratic traditions include:

- Unity between universe, mind, body and spirit
- A universal life force (animal magnetism, bioenergy, chi, pneuma, prana, vis medicatrix naturae)
- Health as the balance and harmony between mind, body and spirit and between living beings and nature
- Disease as the loss of this balance and harmony
- Healers as facilitators, using subtle methods and interventions to stimulate the body's own healing abilities to restore balance, harmony and the free flow of the universal life force.

Functional symptoms and illnesses like IBS provide all of us—people with symptoms, patients with syndromes and doctors who care—with an opportunity to explore and understand the mind-body-spirit connection and its interrelatedness to genetics (heredity) and the environment, both physical (the world around you) and social (your relationship with others and with society).

This new language—this new dialogue—reveals that it is no longer appropriate to separate mind from body, mind from gut or mind-body from spirit. In her book, *Molecules of Emotion,* neuroscientist Candace Pert, Ph.D., has suggested that the term "mind-body" should no longer be hyphenated. John Sarno, M.D., has also endorsed this concept in his book, *The Mindbody Prescription.* We agree and further propose that the most appropriate and inclusive term is "MindBodySpirit." We will use this term in the rest of the book, as you explore the new language of MindBodySpirit in connection with medicine and healing.

*(continued from previous page)*

This notion is also seen in the Far Eastern symbol of yin yang, which becomes the head of our logo figure. This symbol represents the opposing forces that are found in nature, as well as the human spirit. The two opposite forces must work together in order for nature and/or the spirit to be in complete harmony/unity.

The clouds seen behind the Vitruvius figure suggest spirit, which is all encompassing. Spirit is a guiding force as we lead our everyday lives. When mind, body and spirit are in balance, there is a greater possibility of living a happy and healthy life.

– *Michela Ossi*

In the next step, you will begin your journey toward discovering why you are ill and what you can do to help yourself heal by understanding the neuroscience of the MindBodySpirit Connection.

# STEP 2

## UNDERSTANDING THE NEUROBIOLOGY OF THE MINDBODYSPIRIT CONNECTION

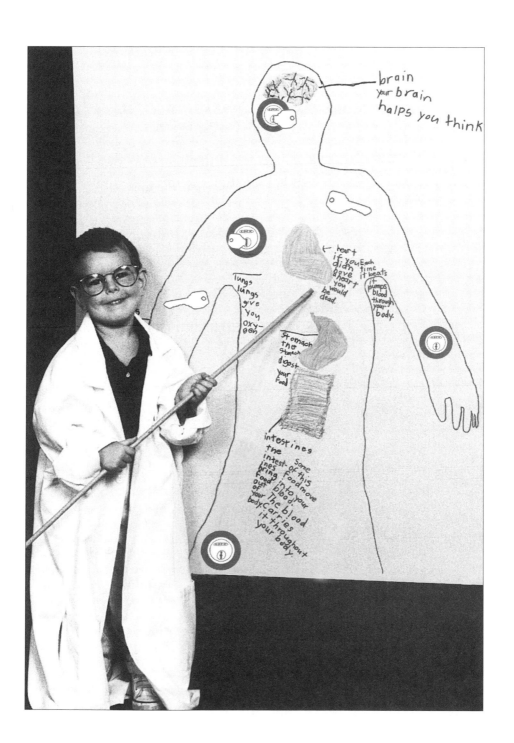

# Chapter 7

## *The MindBodySpirit Connection*

If we're to understand what role our emotions may play
in our health, then understanding the molecular-cellular
domain is the crucial first step.
*– Molecules of Emotion*
Dr. Candace Pert
Neuroscientist

Scientific mechanisms are being unraveled which form the
basis to understand the mechanism(s) of action of mind-body
or complimentary interventions.
– Emeran A. Mayer, M.D.
UCLA Mind-Body Collaborative Research Center,
UCLA School of Medicine
Los Angeles, California

There is a new and comprehensive scientific and neurobiologic
appreciation of the MindBodySpirit Connection and its interrela-
tionship with genetics and the environment, which permits a new
way of understanding irritable bowel syndrome and functional
symptoms/syndromes. Your symptoms are not imagined, psy-
choneurotic, psychosomatic or "all in your head." They are in your
MindBodySpirit Connection!

You have two brains—one in your head and one in your gut—and they
are connected. In fact, they both came from the same part of you when
you were growing as an embryo. You will learn much more about the
"little brain in your gut" and its connection with "the big brain in your

head" in Step 3. For now, we will show you that it is not possible to explain the pain and symptoms of your IBS without understanding the science and neurobiology of your MindBodySpirit Connection.

# The Connection of Mind, Brain, Body and Spirit

You learned about the distinction between mind and brain in Chapter 3. The brain plays the central role of translating the content of your mind—perceptions, thoughts, beliefs, attitudes, hopes, memories, expectations and emotions—into patterns of nerve cell firing and chemical release.

The mind connects with the body by way of three MindBodySpirit communication systems: (1) the central nervous system (CNS), (2) the chemical messenger system (CMS) and (3) the autonomic nervous system (ANS). The three MindBodySpirit communication systems are illustrated in Figure 7.1. There are three sub-systems, called the hypothalamic-pituitary-adrenal axis (HPA axis), the Mind/Brain-Gut Connection and the pain and symptom modulation systems, which are discussed at the end of the chapter.

# The Central Nervous System (CNS)

The CNS is composed of the brain and the spinal cord. The first way that the mind communicates with the rest of the body is by sending messages from the brain through the nerves that branch off of your spine. You are able to move your body, get out of bed, drive to work, play tennis, and so on, when your mind's intention to move is translated by the brain into neurochemicals (see the chemical messenger system for more details) and electrical impulses. The chemical and electrical impulses, through contractions of your skeletal muscles, result in the movement of your body.

In addition to simple muscular activity, your CNS plays a complex role in the orchestration of the MindBodySpirit Connection by way of its connection with the chemical messenger system (CMS) and the autonomic nervous system (ANS). This complex interaction is called the brain neuromatrix.

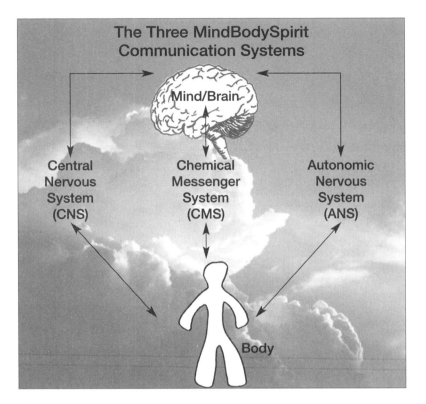

**Figure 7.1**

## The brain neuromatrix

Ronald Melzack is a famous neuroscientist who has described the neuro-matrix of the CNS (*Pain Forum*, 1996;5:125–128). Webster's Dictionary defines matrix as "something within which something else originates or develops." In this sense, the brain neuromatrix represents the complex con-nection of brain cells, nerve impulses and chemical releases within which the mind (perceptions, thoughts, beliefs, feelings and memories) originate or develop. The brain neuromatrix represents the part of our physical brain that translates the invisible mind into visible nerve cell impulses and chem-ical release. It is the conductor of the MindBodySpirit orchestra. The neu-romatrix is composed of several specialized areas, as shown in Figure 7.2:

1.  The **frontal lobes** control thought and cognition. They are located behind your forehead.

## The Neuromatrix

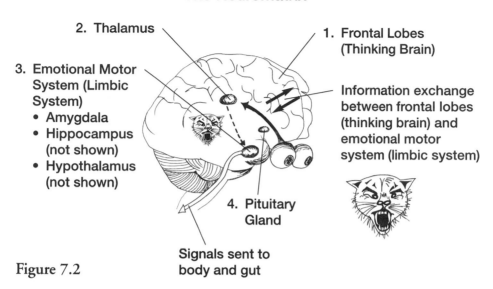

2. Thalamus

1. Frontal Lobes
(Thinking Brain)

3. Emotional Motor
System (Limbic
System)
- Amygdala
- Hippocampus
(not shown)
- Hypothalamus
(not shown)

Information exchange
between frontal lobes
(thinking brain) and
emotional motor
system (limbic system)

4. Pituitary
Gland

Signals sent to
body and gut

Figure 7.2

2. The **thalamus** serves as a switching station for signals sent to and from the brain and body. It is located deep in the center of the brain and is a central relay station for the five senses, with the exception of the olfactory system (responsible for smell), which connects directly to the limbic system.

3. The **limbic system (emotional motor system)** is responsible for the experience and expression of emotion. It is located in the core of the brain and includes the amygdala, hippocampus and hypothalamus.

4. The **pituitary gland** is located at the base of the hypothalamus. It is called the "master gland," since its hormones influence every part of the MindBodySpirit Connection.

The brain neuromatrix represents a "neuro-symphony," where the sounds and rhythms of your thoughts, emotions, hormones, neurochemicals and nerve cell impulses blend into one unified whole. This is the essence of the MindBodySpirit Connection. Let's examine the limbic system in more detail.

### The limbic system (emotional motor system)

In the limbic system, *experience is translated into expression.* The amygdala of the limbic system processes input from all of your sensory systems—vision, touch, hearing, taste and smell. The olfactory system of smell is wired directly into the limbic system. Emotional *experience* is mediated by two-way connections between the amygdala and the frontal lobes (the thinking brain). Your rich inner emotional life depends upon this inter-relationship. The amygdala is the gateway to the limbic system and passes sensory input on to the hypothalamus.

The hypothalamus is the control center of the limbic system and is connected to the pituitary gland and the autonomic nervous system (see later discussion). It is responsible for the bodily *expression* of emotional responses, such as fear and anger. These emotional responses to perceived threat are like computer programs that operate in your defense, helping you to face danger and threat. In his book, *The Emotional Brain: The Mysterious Underpinnings of Emotional Life,* New York University neuro-researcher Joseph LeDoux writes that emotions are hard-wired biologic functions of the CNS that evolved to help animals survive in a hostile environment. Stimulation of this emotional motor system affects every organ of the body through the MindBodySpirit communication systems. This explains how the sight of a threatening tiger can raise your heart rate and blood pressure, cause you to sweat, tighten your muscles and contract your gut. This is how bodily symptoms are related to emotional states of mind.

But emotions and feelings are not the same. You may not know that an emotional response is happening to you. Dr. LeDoux emphasizes that the output of the emotional brain—for example, either an anger or anxiety/fear response to a perceived threat—is not necessarily associated with conscious awareness of anger or anxiety. Thus, a person may exhibit the physiologic signs and symptoms of anxiety but not "feel" anxious. So the gut symptoms of abdominal pain and bowel disturbance that lead to the diagnosis of IBS can be mediated through your emotional motor system without your being aware of anger, anxiety or stress. Learn more about the emotional brain.

Because the emotional motor system often operates at a level that is below conscious awareness, it is important to use your bodily symptoms as a barometer for emotional distress and stress. Even though you may not "feel" distressed, the emotion and stress is in your body and gut. The goal is to move it into conscious awareness, where you can take action to prevent or moderate it. As with all healing, you must learn how to make the invisible workings of your emotional motor system visible to your conscious awareness. By so doing, you will be able to intervene appropriately to maintain health and wellness.

# The Chemical Messenger System (CMS)

The most recently discovered communication system of the MindBody-Spirit Connection is the chemical messenger system. In order to appreciate this system, you will need to understand some basic concepts of cell biology.

## More than the five senses

Like doors and windows in a house, your sensory organs let you interface with the world around you. You already know the five major sense organs of sight, hearing, touch, taste and smell. You may not know that the internal surface of your digestive tract is actually another sense organ—or interface with the outside world—that is actually much larger in surface area than the surface of your skin (see Chapter 11 for more details).

In addition to the major sense organs, every cell in your body has thousands of locations on its surface that serve as "mini" sense organs, called *receptor sites*. These receptor sites are actually proteins that are on the surface of each cell. They act as little receivers (or ears) that listen to the messages of the chemical messenger molecules as they float in the intercellular fluid surrounding every cell. Another way to think of this is to consider each receptor site as a lock that is capable of receiving particular types of chemical messenger keys, called *ligands* (rhymes with "Bye Hands") as illustrated in Figure 7.3.

## Chemical Messenger System

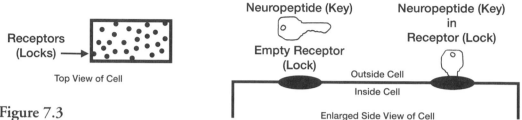

Figure 7.3

There are three different kinds of ligands or chemical messenger keys. They are:

1. neuropeptides (enkephalin, CCK and VIP);
2. neurotransmitters (serotonin and norepinephrine); and
3. steroids (cortisol, testosterone and estrogen).

Figure 7.4 illustrates the chemical messenger communication system found throughout your mind/brain and body. Chemical messenger molecules ("keys") float in your bloodstream and in the fluid that surrounds your cells. The cells contain receptor sites ("locks"). Receptor sites ignore all but the particular type of neuropeptide to which they are attracted. Let's consider just one type of chemical ligand called a neuropeptide. Imagine that a neuropeptide key enters the keyhole of a receptor site. As the key turns inside the lock, the message encoded in the neuropeptide is transmitted to the receptor site, which then opens the cell door to transmit information from the outside surface of the cell to its interior.

Messenger keys function in two different ways, as either agonists or antagonists. When functioning as an agonist, the neuropeptide key fits into the the receptor site lock, turns appropriately and opens the door. Opening the door stimulates the specific action for which the given receptor site is responsible (pain relief, water conservation, sexual arousal, etc.). When functioning as an antagonist, the neuropeptide fits into the keyhole but won't open the lock. In this case, no message is transmitted and the designated action of the receptor site is blocked. The roles of antagonists and agonists will become clearer as you learn about the

Mind/Brain-Gut Connection (Chapter 11) and drug therapies for IBS (Chapter 18).

## Molecules of emotion

In her book, *Molecules of Emotion: Why You Feel the Way You Feel,* Dr. Candace Pert, the neuro-scientist who revolutionized the field of MindBody medicine with her discovery of morphine receptors in the brain, describes how all the cells of the body together form a vast net-work in which all types of infor-mation, including emotional information, is circulated. This network allows organs from different systems—for example, the heart from the cir-culatory system and the liver from the diges-tive system—to influence and affect one another. Messages (and symptoms) coming from one location in your body can reach organs and cells in virtually any other part of your body, like a cell phone that actu-ally works from wherever you happen to be! The existence of this communications network explains how thoughts and feelings can affect virtually every bodily organ. These thoughts and feelings can have a negative or positive effect. For example, a fight with your spouse may increase your abdominal cramping and diarrhea, whereas feelings of hope may actually reduce your abdominal pain.

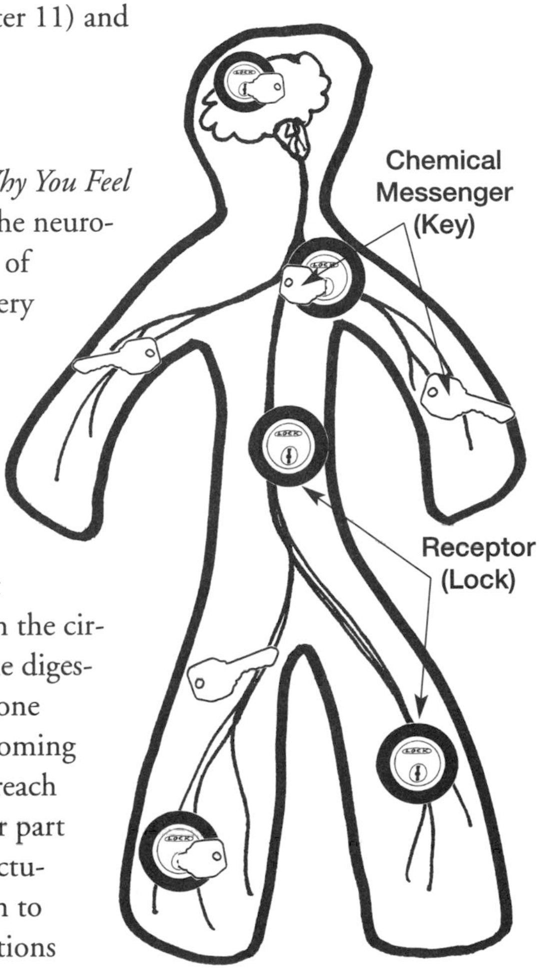

Chemical
Messenger
(Key)

Receptor
(Lock)

**Figure 7.4**

The system works in reverse as well. Pain that originates in the body can affect your mood and behavior. For example, if you develop a sudden and severe abdominal cramp and the urge to go to the bathroom when you are out shopping, considerable anxiety and fear are generated. The body is upsetting the mind.

49

# The Autonomic Nervous System (ANS)

The third MindBodySpirit communication system is the autonomic nervous system, which controls the functioning of the internal organs, including the gut, the glands, the heart and the blood vessels (Figure 7.5). The workings of the autonomic nervous system are for the most part involuntary and automatic. Without your thinking about it, your body maintains the precise functioning of your blood pressure, heart rate, body temperature, respiration, bowel and bladder function and production of saliva, sweat and tears.

The act of breathing bridges the gap between automatic functioning and voluntary control. When you don't think about it, your breathing occurs automatically and unconsciously. When you do think about it, you can control your breathing. Breathing techniques have been used for thousands of years as an essential element in virtually every meditative technique or healing practice. You will learn more about the importance of conscious breathing as a relaxation technique later in this book.

There are two branches of the autonomic nervous system—the sympathetic branch and the parasympathetic branch—which act in opposition

## Autonomic Nervous System (ANS)

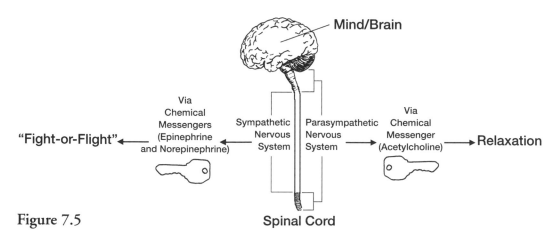

Figure 7.5

to each other. For example, when the sympathetic branch is activated in response to stressors, the parasympathetic branch is inactive, or suppressed. When the parasympathetic branch is activated, the sympathetic branch is suppressed.

Both branches of the ANS originate from the hypothalamus of the emotional motor system of the CNS. They branch out to interface with virtually every organ, blood vessel and sweat gland in your body. The ANS, for example, is at work when a scary event causes your hair to stand on end. When a fear signal is sent from your mind/brain down the "wires" of your ANS, little muscles at the base of each hair follicle are stimulated to raise your hair! Goosebumps occur by the same mechanism. Let's examine the two branches in more detail.

## The sympathetic branch of the ANS

The nerves that control the sympathetic branch of the ANS originate in the thoracic (chest) and lumbar (lower back) segments of the spinal cord. The sympathetic nervous system is activated during emergencies—or what you perceive or interpret to be emergencies. You become alert, vigilant, aroused, activated and prepared for action.

The sympathetic branch uses the neuropeptides epinephrine (also called adrenaline) and norepinephrine (also called noradrenaline) to activate your body's "fight or flight" stress response. Epinephrine and norepinephrine are collectively called "catecholamines." You can see epinephrine and norepinephrine as the "key" that leads to "fight or flight" in Figure 7.5. When you have a "near miss" in your car, it is your sympathetic nervous system—releasing epinephrine from your adrenal glands and norepinephrine from sympathetic nerve endings—that causes you to be tremulous, sweaty and to feel that clutching sensation in your gut.

## The parasympathetic branch of the ANS

The parasympathetic branch of the ANS has nerve fibers that originate in the cranial (top) and sacral (bottom) segments of the spinal cord. The parasympathetic branch calms the body, which is the precise opposite of the sympathetic branch. The parasympathetic system promotes routine activities, such as digesting your food. It slows the heart rate, whereas the sympathetic system speeds it up. It sends blood to the digestive tract, while the sympathetic system sends it to the muscles. The parasympathetic nervous system secretes the neurochemical acetylcholine, which is the "key" leading to relaxation (Figure 7.5). The lowering of heart rate and blood pressure and the reduction of muscle tension are produced by the parasympathetic branch. Stress management techniques aim to induce a positive parasympathetic state.

Safety features are built into your body to prevent the sympathetic and parasympathetic nervous systems from simultaneously activating, just as cars have safety features to prevent you from pressing on both the gas and brake pedals at the same time. For this reason, your body is usually either in a sympathetic (stressed) state or a parasympathetic (relaxed) state.

## Sub-Systems of the MindBodySpirit Communication Systems

Three important sub-systems function within the MindBodySpirit communication systems. The connection of the hypothalamus, pituitary gland and adrenal glands, called the "HPA Axis," will be discussed in the next chapter (Chapter 8). The Mind/Brain-Gut Connection will be described in Chapter 11. The third sub-system, the pain and symptom modulation system, is discussed here.

The MindBodySpirit Connection has communication sub-systems for the regulation and control of pain that doctors and scientists call "pain modulation systems." Although they are somewhat complex, we will focus upon two of them: the gate control process and endorphins.

### The gate control process

The mind can modify the experience and feeling of bodily pain and symptoms. Signals coming up the spinal cord—from the body to the brain—can either be enhanced or blocked through the descending inhibitory pathway of the "gate control" process, illustrated in Figure 7.6. Dr. Melzack, who recently modified his model to include the neuromatrix of the CNS discussed earlier, initially described this process. For

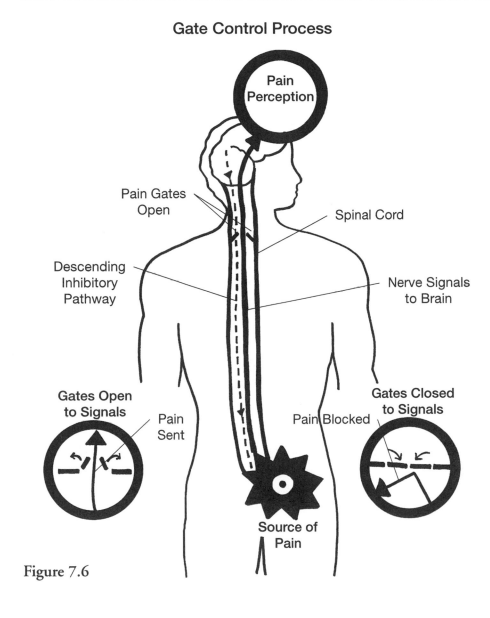

**Figure 7.6**

example, concentrating on something other than the pain—working hard, playing a sport or watching a movie—can "close the gate" to the sensation of pain as the mind/brain sends a blocking message down the inhibitory pathway. By contrast, you can "open the gate" to pain by impeding the blocking message, thus increasing the experience of the pain. Depression can open the gate and enhance pain, as can negative thinking and beliefs. You will learn how to close the gate to pain later in this book.

## Endorphins

The second pain modulation system in the body involves internal pain-killing neuropeptides called endorphins. Endorphins are part of your chemical messenger system (CMS) and they represent a form of internally created morphine-like pain relievers. They block pain by binding to opioid (morphine) receptor sites in the brain and body, where they turn off the pain signal (Figure 7.7). Candace Pert, who first discovered these receptor sites, tells the exciting story of her discovery in her book, *Molecules of Emotion.*

**Figure 7.7**

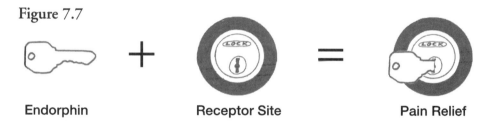

Endorphin                     Receptor Site                     Pain Relief

In the next chapter, you will see how the "good stress" response helps you to maintain an inner balance and stability called homeostasis.

# Chapter 8
## *"Good Stress" Response*

... the unpleasant or potentially harmful things happening
in the environment are referred to as stressors, while the
psychological and biological reactions they elicit are referred
to as the stress response.
    – *The Healing Mind*
    Paul Martin, Ph.D.


Allostasis—the ability to achieve stability (homeostasis)
through change—is critical to survival.
    – Bruce S. McEwen, Ph.D.,
    Neuroendocrinologist,
    The Rockefeller University, New York


Stressors (triggers) are anything that throws the MindBodySpirit
Connection out of balance (homeostasis). When your mind/brain
interprets stressors (triggers) to be a threat to internal balance and
harmony, then a protective "good stress" response is generated in
order to restore homeostasis. Allostasis is the process of achieving
stability (homeostasis) through change, which operates by way of
the MindBodySpirit communication systems. Allostasis is crucial for
your health and survival.


The term *stress* is generally considered to be equivalent to *psychological*
stress in response to external stressors or triggers. Furthermore, psychological stress (mind) is usually considered to be fundamentally separate
from the "real" biological factors (body) that underlie disease and illness.
But there is a new scientific appreciation that stress, mind, body and

spirit are interconnected and interrelated with genetics and the environment and that understanding this will help you to heal from your IBS and live a healthy life.

# Homeostasis: Internal Balance

For centuries, and in all societies, people with medical problems have turned to healers who helped them recognize their own innate healing capabilities through achieving internal harmony and balance. The wisdom of ancient, traditional and modern comprehensive approaches to health, healing and disease has been confirmed by new scientific understandings of this internal harmony and balance called homeostasis. Certain bodily systems, such as blood oxygen, acid-base status (or pH) and body temperature must be maintained within fairly narrow ranges, and your MindBodySpirit Connection does this automatically in health. But you must also be able to respond to stress, such as changes in your physical states (awake, asleep, lying down, standing up, exercising) and coping with threats (danger, infection, temperature extremes, noise, loss, overcrowding, isolation and hunger). Homeostasis is the process of maintaining balance in the face of this constant change.

# Stress

Like most people, you probably think of stress as something that happens to you, which makes you feel stressed. But in his book on stress, stress-related diseases and coping entitled *Why Zebras Don't Get Ulcers,* Robert M. Sapolsky, Ph.D., Professor of Biological Sciences and Neurosciences, Stanford University, says that, "A *stressor* can be defined as anything that throws your body out of *allostatic balance*—for example, an injury, subjection to great heat or cold. The *stress response,* in turn, is your body's attempt to restore balance. This consists of the secretion of certain hormones, the inhibition of others, the activation of particular parts of the nervous system, and other physiologic changes . . ." Let's look at *stressors, stress response* and *allostatic balance (allostasis)* more closely.

# Stressors (Triggers)

Stressors/triggers take many forms and can be either physical and real (tangible and measurable)—what we call *"the tiger in your path,"* or they can be perceived and interpreted (intangible and immeasurable)—what we call *"the tiger in your mind."* Some examples of stressors/triggers are listed in Table 8.1.

Table 8.1

### Potential Stressors/Triggers

| Physical and Real *"The Tiger in Your Path"* | Perceived and Interpreted *"The Tiger in Your Mind"* |
|---|---|
| • Temperature extremes | • Social (home, neighborhood, work, interpersonal) |
| • Circadian light-dark cycle | |
| • Seasonal change | • Major life events |
| • Travel ("jet lag") | • Trauma, abuse |
| • Accident | • Loss (death, divorce, job loss) |
| • Injury | • Anxiety |
| • Inflammation | • Depression |
| • Infection | |
| • Poisons/toxins | |
| • Food | |
| • Medications | |
| • Surgery | |
| • Menstruation | |
| • Menopause | |
| • Medical disease | |

## Stressors: External, internal or both

Emeran A. Mayer, a gastroenterologist and Director of the UCLA Mind Body Collaborative Research Center, says that "Stress, defined as acute threats to the homeostasis of an organism, be they real (physical) or perceived (psychological), and whether posed by events in the *outside* world or from *within,* evokes adaptive responses which serve to defend the stability of the internal environment and to assure the survival of the organism"

(*Gut,* 2000;47:861–869 and *The Biological Basis for Mind-Body Interactions,* volume 6, 122 edn. Amsterdam: Elsevier Science, 2000). A stressor can be *external, internal* or both *external and internal.*

## Stress Response

Although some stressors/triggers may be difficult to classify as physical, perceived, external or internal, it is vital to distinguish *stressors* from the *stress response* they elicit within the MindBodySpirit Connection and to understand the adaptive process called *allostasis.* In his book, *The Healing Mind,* Dr. Paul Martin writes, "The unpleasant or potentially harmful things happening in the environment are referred to as stressors, while the psychological and biological reactions they elicit are referred to as the stress response."

## Allostasis: The Good Stress Response

Most likely—until now—you have never heard the terms *allostasis* and *allostatic load,* but they are terms that we hope you will understand and appreciate for the rest of your life. Dr. Bruce McEwen, in the January 15, 1998, issue of the *New England Journal of Medicine,* introduced the term *allostasis,* which comes from the Greek words "allo" (meaning variable) and "stasis" (meaning stability). Thus, allostasis represents the dynamic and variable processes used by the MindBodySpirit Connection to achieve and maintain homeostasis. Allostasis is critical for your survival and good health.

As Dr. McEwen says, the "good stress" response of allostasis is protective and restorative. It allows your MindBodySpirit Connection to maintain homeostasis in the face of stressors/triggers (Figure 8.1). Major stressors (such as the loss of a loved one, divorce or loss of a job) as well as minor stressors (the daily wear and tear of living, family arguments or being stopped in a traffic jam) set off the release of stress hormones that boost your body's level of alertness and energy in order to help your MindBodySpirit Connection meet the challenge. "During episodes of

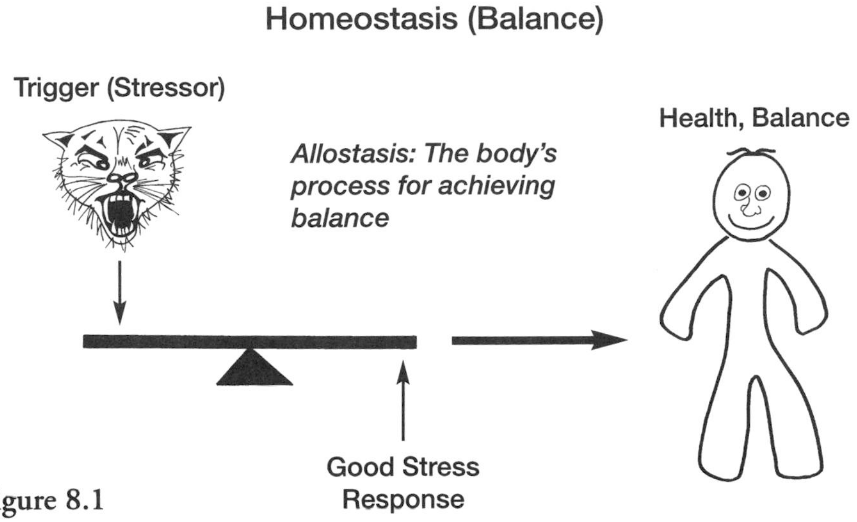

**Homeostasis (Balance)**

Trigger (Stressor)

*Allostasis: The body's process for achieving balance*

Health, Balance

**Good Stress Response**

Figure 8.1

acute stress, stress hormones provide a protective function by activating the body's defenses," says Dr. McEwen. Let's take a look at how the good stress response works to protect and restore your homeostasis through allostasis.

# How the Good Stress Response Works Through the HPA

When homeostasis is threatened by a stressor/trigger, the limbic system (emotional motor system) is activated (see Chapter 7). Remember that the limbic system contains computer-like programs for your defense. The hypothalamus of the limbic system sends chemical and nerve signals to the pituitary gland, which then communicates with the adrenal glands that sit on top of the kidneys. This linkage is called the hypothalamic-pituitary-adrenal axis (HPA), which is one of the subsystems of the MindBodySpirit communication systems described in Chapter 7. Some of the signals sent through the HPA activate certain glands or organs and some of the signals inhibit or suppress certain glands or organs. This is the initial step of the stress response. There are two parallel pathways that emerge from the HPA, the epinephrine pathway and the cortisol pathway.

## The epinephrine pathway

The first pathway of your stress response system activates within seconds, when the sympathetic branches of the autonomic nervous system carry the alarm signal from the hypothalamus of the limbic system to the adrenal medulla (the inner portion of the adrenal gland), which releases epinephrine. Recall that epinephrine is one of two catecholamines released by the activation of the sympathetic nervous system. The other is norepinephrine. Epinephrine prepares the body for quick action. Blood flow shifts from the skin and digestive tract to the muscles, your heart rate increases, your blood pressure rises and you become more alert.

## The cortisol pathway

The second pathway of your stress response system activates over the course of minutes or hours, when the hypothalamus secretes several hormones and neurochemicals into the HPA axis. The main chemical released—CRF, or corticotropin releasing factor—is secreted within 15 seconds and triggers the pituitary to release the hormone ACTH (adreno-corticotropic hormone). ACTH then travels via the blood stream as part of the chemical messenger system, through which it reaches the adrenal glands. Within several minutes, ACTH stimulates the adrenal cortex (the outer part of the adrenal gland) to release cortisol. Cortisol increases blood sugar for energy. Cortisol also feeds back to the pituitary to turn off the release of CRF, thereby slowing down the responses initiated by epinephrine. Cortisol also acts on the brain to improve your ability to remember events related to the stress.

As you can see, the good stress response is remarkably complex, much like a conductor leading an orchestra of nerve cells, glands, smooth muscles and neurochemicals. The conductor (the brain neuromatrix) must orchestrate the subtle movement of every gland, muscle, nerve cell fiber and organ system in the body—leading some to play loudly, while others wait silently for their turn.

The good stress response is also known as the "fight-or-flight" response, since it is designed for your protection. The relaxation response, on the other hand, is associated with a decrease in the very same chemical messengers that cause the fight-or-flight response. You will learn how to elicit the relaxation response later in this book.

# Variability of the Stress Response

Exposed to the same trigger/stressor, people vary remarkably in their stress response. For example, for some women, menstruation is an internal stressor that produces a dramatic and powerful stress response in their mind, body and spirit. For other women, the same stressor/trigger hardly produces any bodily or emotional response at all. Another example is that most—but not all—people find that public speaking is very stressful, even just the thought or anticipation of it. Dr. McEwen points out that there are two factors that account for this variability of the stress response—the way a person perceives a situation and a person's general state of physical health. Thus, your mind/brain may or may not consider public speaking to be a potential threat to your homeostasis, so the stress response may or may not be activated. If your general health is good, you will be more likely to tolerate your stress response than if you are in poor health. Your physical health is also affected by heredity (IBS, heart disease or high blood pressure in the family), your lifestyle choices (smoking, underexercising, eating a high fat diet), your psychological choices (unresolved anger, excessive worry) and your spiritual choices (sense of meaning or purpose in life, connection to a higher power). Your physical condition and how well you care for yourself play a critical role in influencing your stress response.

Learn more about <u>allostasis and the good stress response</u>.

# The Good and the Bad

Allostasis and the "good stress" response protect us. Robert Sapolsky, Professor of Biological Sciences and Neuroscience at Stanford University, says, "Allostasis refers to the notion that different circumstances demand different homeostatic set points (after all, the ideal blood pressure when you are sleeping is likely to be quite different than when you are bungee-jumping), and that maintaining whatever an optimal set point might be typically demands far-flung regulatory changes throughout the body instead of just local adjustments." Many people actually seek out the "good stress" response—by riding on roller-coasters, sky diving, bungee jumping and participating in "extreme" sports.

The good stress response turns on in response to a stressor/trigger, such as a dangerous situation, an infection or having to speak in public. It turns off when the danger has passed, when the infection is controlled or when the speech has been given. However, if the turn-on and turn-off systems malfunction, the MindBodySpirit Connection can be overexposed to the stress response hormones. In this way, over weeks, months and years, the good stress response can turn bad and make you sick with what Dr. MeEwen calls *allostatic load.*

This price that we pay for the ability to adapt to stressors/triggers—allostatic load—is the lesson of the next chapter.

# Chapter 9
## "Bad Stress" Response

From the standpoint of health, what is even more important than how we feel about the stressful events in our lives is how our bodies react in terms of the stress hormones they produce.
— Bruce S. McEwen, Ph.D., Neuroscientist

Alterations in the responsiveness of this system (the bad stress response) on a genetic basis or due to environmental influences, are important factors in the pathophysiology of a wide range of chronic diseases ranging from coronary artery (ischemic) heart disease to irritable bowel syndrome.
— Emeran A. Mayer, M.D.,
UCLA Mind Body Collaborative Research Center,
Los Angeles, California

Stress, it's the biggest killer on the planet.
— Willie Nelson (singer)

The stress response of the MindBodySpirit Connection may or may not be associated with the conscious experience of fear or anxiety. The perception of stress varies from person to person, and over the long run, your good stress response may turn bad, which burdens your mind, body and spirit with what scientists call allostatic load. This results in an imbalance and disturbance of homeostasis within the MindBodySpirit Connection that can result in functional symptoms. Collections of these symptoms commonly lead to the diagnosis of IBS and other functional syndromes. Even worse, this imbalance and disturbance can contribute to the development of serious diseases, such as metabolic syndrome X, which can kill you.

## Stressed Out?

What does it mean to be "stressed out"? Does it mean having a bad day? Is it having a fight with your family or getting criticized by your boss? Is it feeling bummed out or frazzled? Most people look at only the short-term consequences of stress. However, it's the long-term consequences of your stress response that burden your MindBodySpirit Connection with a load that can make you sick.

# There's a Tiger in Your Path

The body's stress response system—mediated through the HPA axis and the secretion of epinephrine and cortisol—was really designed to handle short term, life threatening, physical survival risks. If you were really being chased by a raging tiger, you would be grateful to have the fight-or-flight good stress response on your side. Its nerve cell firing and chemical messengers would mobilize release of energy from storage sites to supply contracting muscles, increase heart rate and blood pressure in order to circulate blood throughout the body and suppress functions not necessary for your immediate survival, such as digestion. Survival is more important than digesting your lunch!

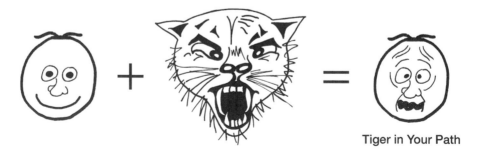

**Tiger in Your Path**

# There's a Tiger in Your Mind

In today's world, the fight-or-flight good stress response is most commonly turned on by stressors that are neither short term, life threatening, nor a risk to your physical survival. Today's tiger is usually *not* in your path, but in your mind—everyday worries, hustles, hassles and strains. These "tigers in your mind" activate your fight-or-flight response in ways identical to the stress response that would be activated by real live tigers.

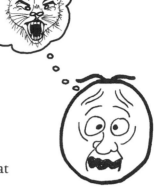

Tiger in Your Mind

The long term consequences of these "tigers in the mind" are many and varied and lead to overactivation of the stress response. Let's look at the origins of these "tigers in the mind."

## The past

You repeatedly recall a previous life event that was stressful to you, such as an auto accident, a bad relationship or an unfortunate misunderstanding. When severe, recurrent and unstoppable memories of past stressful events trigger the stress response, it is called Post-Traumatic Stress Disorder, or PTSD.

## The present

You hurt your back while working in the yard. In addition to the physical pain, you are afraid that you may miss work and be unable to pay your bills or care for your family. Your fear, anger, frustration and anxiety are "tigers in the mind."

Your imagination may also be a "tiger in the mind." For example, you may think that someone is trying to harm you or your reputation, even though it is not true.

## The future

You have a big speech to give next month in front of a lot of people. You can't get it off of your mind. You become what Joan Borysenko, Ph.D., calls an "advanced worrier." Your excessive worry is a "tiger in the mind."

# "But I Don't Feel Stressed": The Crouching Tiger

You might be thinking, "This is all very interesting, but I don't feel stressed or anxious, so none of this could be related to my IBS symptoms." But the reality is that the stress response may be activated without any conscious awareness of feeling stressed. We call this "the crouching tiger in the mind"—when your stress response is activated but you don't feel stressed.

Dr. Joseph LeDoux, neuroscientist at New York University, discusses the impact of emotion on the MindBodySpirit in his book, *The Emotional Brain: The Mysterious Underpinnings of Emotional Life.* He says that the triggers/stressors of the stress response are not necessarily perceived or realized. The physical expression of the stress response—for example, the symptoms of IBS—are not necessarily accompanied by a mental awareness of anxiety, fear or stress. So you can have the abdominal pain and bowel function disturbances of IBS without feeling nervous or stressed. Learn more about the emotional brain.

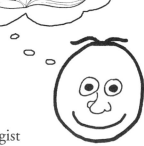

Crouching Tiger

Furthermore, psychological tests for anxiety may be normal despite activation of the emotional motor system within the brain neuromatrix. In other words, you would not necessarily be found to have "abnormal" anxiety or fear were you to be evaluated by a psychologist or psychiatrist or to take a psychological test.

# The "Bad Stress" Response

You have learned that your MindBodySpirit Connection has been designed with elaborate communication systems that orchestrate a coordinated response to stressors/triggers. This ability to defend homeostasis (that is, to maintain internal stability and balance) through change is called *allostasis*.

In a healthy person, the communication and response systems are turned on and off rapidly so that the "good stress" response is synchronized with the duration of the trigger. Your exposure to the potentially harmful effects of the stress response is limited, and homeostasis is restored.

But there are several situations in which the severity or chronicity of the stressor/trigger can cause a "bad stress" response that aggravates existing disease processes or predisposes you to the development of new ones. In other words, allostasis becomes maladaptive rather than adaptive. The MindBodySpirit Connection becomes imbalanced and disturbed (see Figure 9.1). Dr. McEwen says, "During episodes of acute stress, stress hormones provide a protective function by activating the body's defenses, but when these same protective hormones are produced repeatedly, or in excess, because of chronic stress, they create a gradual and steady cascade of harmful physiological changes. From the standpoint of health," Dr. McEwen adds, "What is even more important than how we feel about the stressful events in our lives is how our bodies react in terms of the stress hormones they produce." The long-term and harmful effects of the "bad stress" response is called *allostatic load,* which is the wear and tear that results from chronic overactivity or underactivity of the stress response systems operating through the three MindBodySpirit communication systems.

## Disturbed Homeostasis (Imbalance)

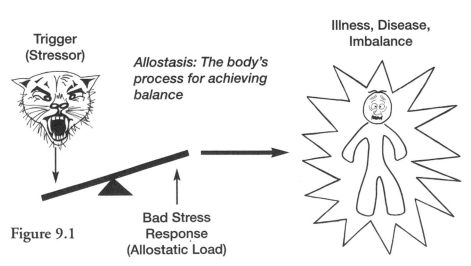

**Trigger (Stressor)**

*Allostasis: The body's process for achieving balance*

**Illness, Disease, Imbalance**

Figure 9.1

**Bad Stress Response (Allostatic Load)**

# The Cost of Allostatic Load

Gastroenterologist Emeran A. Mayer, M.D., of the University of California, Los Angeles (UCLA) Mind-Body Collaborative Research Center, says, "Alterations in the responsiveness of this (stress response) system, on a genetic basis or due to environmental influences, are important factors in the pathophysiology of a wide range of chronic diseases ranging from coronary artery (ischemic) heart disease to irritable bowel syndrome." Some of the most important examples of the harmful effects of the "bad stress" response are listed here.

- Elevations of blood fats, such as cholesterol and triglycerides, that increase the risk of developing atherosclerosis (hardening and narrowing of the arteries).
- Atherosclerosis and high blood pressure (hypertension) leading to arterial blood vessel problems that include circulation impairment, heart disease and stroke. In his book, *Why Zebras Don't Get Ulcers,* Stanford's Robert Sapolsky says, "If your blood pressure rises to 180/120 when you are sprinting away from a lion, you are being adaptive, but if it is 180/120 every time you see a mess in your teenager's bedroom, you could be headed for a cardiovascular disaster."
- Metabolic Syndrome X. This is the term coined by Stanford's Gerald M. Reaven, M.D. In his books, *Syndrome X: Overcoming the Silent Killer That Can Give You a Heart Attack* and *Syndrome X, the Silent Killer: The New Heart Disease Risk,* Dr. Reaven discusses this metabolic disturbance associated with insulin resistance that interferes with the body's ability to move glucose into cells. Metabolic Syndrome X greatly increases the risk of developing blood vessel disease that can lead to heart disease, stroke and kidney failure. Learn more about Metabolic Syndrome X.

    Metabolic Syndrome X is characterized by:
    - Central obesity (excessive fat in the abdominal area). "People end up with that 'apple' body shape that researchers have shown over and over again predisposes us to heart disease," says Dr. McEwen.
    - Glucose intolerance or diabetes
    - Hypertension

- Hyperlipidemia (elevated blood cholesterol, low HDL cholesterol, high LDL cholesterol and/or elevated triglycerides)
- Suppression of the immune system, which increases vulnerability to infection and certain types of cancer
- Bone damage and weakness that contributes to fractures
- Muscle weakening and loss
- Depression
- Memory loss and actual brain damage
- Functional symptoms and syndromes
- Gastrointestinal disease processes, including inflammatory bowel disease (ulcerative colitis and Crohn's disease), peptic ulcer disease, gastroesophageal reflux disease (GERD), fatty liver and functional gut syndromes, such as IBS. This is why you are reading this book.

# The MindBodySpirit Model of the Bad Stress Response

You are now equipped to understand the neurobiological basis for the functional symptoms discussed in Chapter 1 that lead to the diagnosis of functional syndromes, such as IBS, described in Chapter 2. Refer to the "MindBodySpirit Model of Bad Stress Response" shown in Figure 9.2 as you read the following explanation. Then you will be prepared to learn about IBS and other functional gut symptoms and syndromes in Step 3.

## Genetics and early life experiences

Genetic factors or early life events can alter the responsiveness of the MindBodySpirit Connection to stressors/triggers and the ability to adapt through allostasis, which renders a person susceptible to the bad stress response throughout life. Examples of genetic factors include inherited weaknesses in various body systems. For example, if your father has high blood pressure, then your chances for developing hypertension are increased. Another is that IBS and fibromyalgia tend to run in families.

Here are examples of early life events that increase vulnerability to the bad stress response through allostatic load.

# MindBodySpirit Model of Bad Stress Response (Allostatic Load)

MindBodySpirit Modifying Factors: Spirituality, Faith and Hope; Sharing and Expressing Your Feelings; Changing the Meaning of an Event (Changing Your Thoughts, Feelings, Attitudes or Beliefs); Healthy Lifestyle Choices and Behavior; Medication and Other Treatments

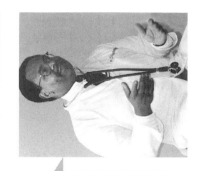

Symptoms and Disease

Doctor/Patient Relationship, Diagnosis, Education, Treatment

Psychological Distress

Neuromatrix

"Bad Stress" Response and Disturbed MindBodySpirit Connection

Perceived Threat to Homeostasis

Genetics and Early Life Experiences

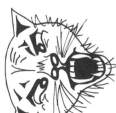

Stressors/ Triggers

Symptom Expression Through MindBodySpirit Communication Systems

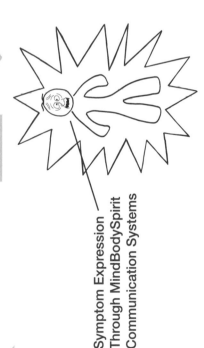

Figure 9.2

- Early life stress in the form of a disrupted and/or disturbed relationship with your primary caregiver (for example, with your mother or father)
- Chronic abuse, either emotional, physical or sexual
- Neglect throughout life
- Loss, such as the death of a parent
- Exposure to a one-time stressor/trigger that is perceived as life threatening (for example, rape, combat, physical trauma, natural disaster). In the most extreme form, this is called Post Traumatic Stress Disorder (PTSD).

Awareness of these predisposing factors can help you to modify their adverse effects upon your mind, body and spirit.

## Stressors/triggers

Reversible alterations in allostatic systems that aggravate symptoms can occur with the many stressors/triggers described in Chapter 8, especially when the stressors/triggers are sustained and perceived as threatening. Examples of this include:

- Losses (divorce, death, job loss)
- Interpersonal distress
- Financial difficulties
- Spiritual distress (loss of meaning, crisis of faith)

Remember that the stress response may not be associated with conscious awareness or feeling of stress or anxiety. This helps explain why functional gut symptoms may vary in severity from time to time, and why the symptoms that you experience may vary. For example, you may have lots of lower abdominal pain associated with constipation, diarrhea or both for a week or longer, and then have the symptoms lessen or disappear for a while.

Your symptoms can also migrate from one body system to another, or from one part of the gut to another. For example, you may experience gut symptoms for months or years, only to find that—one day—these symptoms lessen, and new, different symptoms arise in their place, such as those of fibromyalgia (widespread aching, pain and fatigue). Or IBS symptoms may be replaced by functional dyspepsia, which is pain or discomfort centered in the upper abdomen.

### Perceived threat to homeostasis

Remember that the activation of your stress response system is always accompanied by some perceived threat. In other words, some part of your mind/brain, body or spirit must interpret or perceive a stressor/trigger as a potential threat to your internal balance (homeostasis) before your stress response is activated. Again, the perception of threat may be happening at an unconscious level, where you are not aware of it. Now you see why the process of making the invisible visible—that is, of bringing the unconscious parts of your life into conscious awareness—is so vital to all forms of healing: physical, mental, emotional and spiritual. Unless you become aware of perceived threats and the potential harmful consequences of your bad stress response, you may not be able to heal and become healthy.

## "Bad Stress Response" and the MindBodySpirit Connection

The burden that results from the allostatic load of chronic exposure to the "bad stress" response alters the homeostatic mechanisms. The Mind-BodySpirit communication systems become imbalanced and disturbed, including the pain modulation systems (pain and discomfort), the autonomic nervous system (gut spasm, muscle tension, high blood pressure), the HPA axis (fatigue, sleep disturbance, altered immunity) and psychological distress (heightened awareness of and attention to symptoms, anxiety, depression). This is also why researchers can detect changes in certain chemical messengers, such as serotonin and Substance P (a neurotransmitter), in patients who suffer with functional syndromes. The same underlying imbalance and disturbance of the MindBodySpirit Connection explains the "irritable body syndrome" described in the book's introduction.

Excessive allostatic load from "bad stress" can alter the pain and symptom processing systems of the MindBodySpirit Connection in the same way that loud and distorted sound can damage hearing. Put another way, excess allostatic load disables the mechanisms that exist within your body to modulate pain. As a consequence, even tiny pain signals that would ordinarily not be felt become magnified within the body and cause significant pain. For example, in IBS patients, a small amount of intestinal activity—activity that would not ordinarily be felt—becomes magnified until it is experienced as unpleasant and severe.

Remember—it works both ways. Symptoms in the mind can also be generated from symptoms in the body. For example, increasing pain and cramping from an intestinal infection can stimulate the limbic system, leading to increased emotional arousal in the form of anxiety, fear and hypervigilance.

## Patient-caregiver relationship, diagnosis and education

You can see that the relationship that you have with your doctor or caregiver can affect your symptom experience, as can your diagnosis and whether you really understand your condition and what is happening to you. We will have more to say about this later in the book.

Learn more about <u>allostatic load and the bad stress response</u>.

Take the next step to understand IBS and other functional gut symptoms and syndromes in a new way that will prepare you for healing.

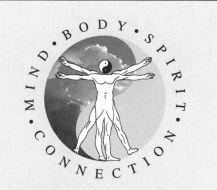

There are actions that you can take to modify the bad stress response and limit its damaging effects on your mind, body and spirit. These are called "Mind-BodySpirit modifying factors." The most important MindBody-Spirit modifying factors include:

- Experiencing spirituality, faith and hope
- Sharing and expressing your feelings
- Changing the meaning of an event, usually by changing your thoughts, feelings, attitudes and beliefs about it
- Making healthy lifestyle choices and behavior (for example, in the areas of diet, exercise and stress management)
- Using medication and other appropriate treatments

You will learn more about these factors in Steps 4, 5, 6 and 7.

# STEP 3

## FOCUSING ON IBS

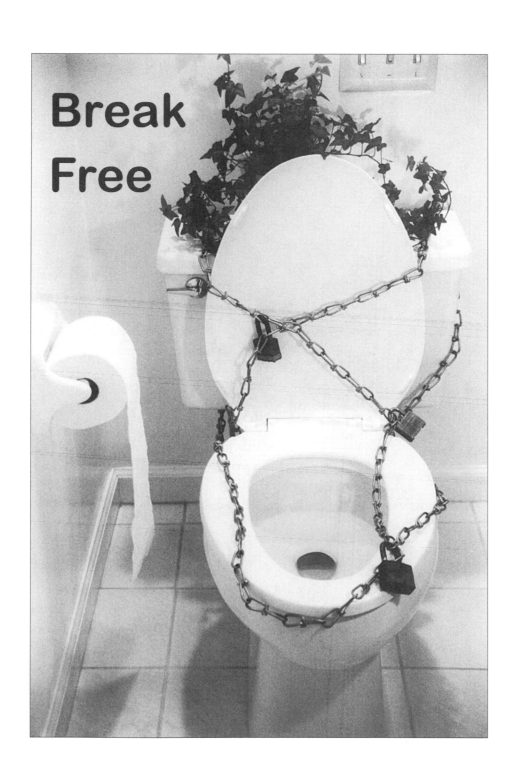

# Chapter 10

## *Gut Anatomy and Physiology*

A healthy body is a guest-chamber for the soul;
a sick body is a prison.
– *The Advancement of Learning*
Sir Francis Bacon

> Do you remember the anatomy and physiology of the gut (gastro-intestinal tract) that you learned in high school health class? If not, here is your lesson again! The gut has five parts and five sphincters (Figure 10.1). The sphincters serve as gateways between the parts.

## The Five Parts of the Gut

The gut has five parts, each of which performs a specific function in the movement, breakdown, digestion, storage and elimination of waste. Food moves through the digestive system by means of powerful, wavelike muscle contractions called peristalsis. The symptoms of IBS are expressed in the fifth part, the colon.

### 1. Mouth and pharynx

The digestive process begins in the mouth. The salivary glands in the cheeks and under the tongue make digestive enzymes called *amylase* and *lipase.* Amylase breaks down starch; lipase breaks down fat. Although it appears to be a simple process, the act of swallowing is actually amazingly complex, involving the simultaneous coordination, contraction and relaxation of dozens of nerves and muscles. Swallowing delivers food to the esophagus through the upper esophageal sphincter.

# The Gastrointestinal Tract

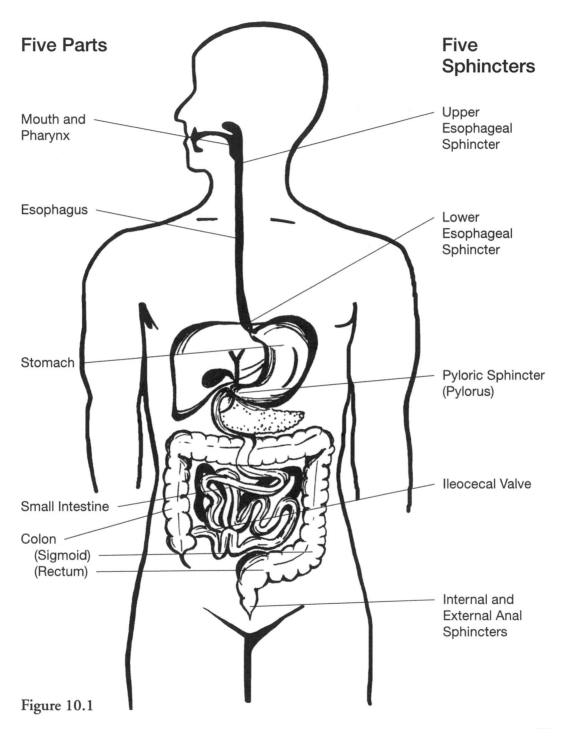

**Five Parts**

Mouth and Pharynx

Esophagus

Stomach

Small Intestine

Colon
(Sigmoid)
(Rectum)

**Five Sphincters**

Upper Esophageal Sphincter

Lower Esophageal Sphincter

Pyloric Sphincter (Pylorus)

Ileocecal Valve

Internal and External Anal Sphincters

Figure 10.1

## 2. Esophagus

The esophagus is a tube about one foot long. It is lined with powerful circular and longitudinal muscles that move swallowed food into the stomach by forceful peristaltic contractions. When the food reaches the end of the esophagus, it passes through the lower esophageal sphincter (LES). The LES is a muscular door that opens and closes, allowing food to enter the stomach from the esophagus while simultaneously preventing the acidic contents of the stomach from coming back up into the esophagus. Esophageal muscle contractions (esophageal peristalsis) are so powerful that if you swallowed food while standing on your head, the esophagus would still transport it to the stomach!

## 3. Stomach

The stomach serves as a temporary holding area for the food. It is here that food is churned, processed and broken down into smaller food particles that can later be absorbed by the small intestine. Food is broken down both physically and chemically. Peristaltic contractions of the stomach physically break down the food into smaller particles. Potent digestive enzymes along with hydrochloric acid (manufactured by the cells in the stomach lining) chemically break down the food.

The stomach empties different foods at different rates. For example, fat takes longer to leave the stomach than other foods, sometimes remaining in the stomach for up to six hours. Liquids empty quickly, often leaving the stomach within 20 to 30 minutes. Usually, most of a regular-sized meal empties from the stomach within two hours. When the food in the stomach is ready for release, it passes through another muscular "door" called the pyloric sphincter, which opens into the first part of the small intestine.

## 4. Small intestine

The small intestine is 15 to 20 feet long and includes three sections: (1) the *duodenum* (which makes up the first 10 inches of the small intestine), (2) the *jejunum* (which makes up the next 5 feet) and (3) the *ileum* (which makes up the rest). Digestion and absorption of food take place primarily in the small intestine.

In the duodenum, bile and pancreatic juice are added to the food mixture. In the jejunum, fat, starch and proteins from the food material are broken down and absorbed by the intestinal lining. The lining is covered with millions of tiny villi, or finger-like projections, that greatly increase the surface area, allowing nutrients to be more efficiently absorbed into the bloodstream. In the ileum, which is the last part of the small intestine, water and nutrients (such as vitamin B12) are absorbed. Bile, which is released by the gallbladder into the duodenum in order to help emulsify (digest) ingested fats, is reabsorbed in the ileum to prevent its loss from the body. As swallowed food and nutrients leave the ileum to enter the large intestine (colon), they pass through another muscular door, the ileocecal valve.

## 5.  Large intestine (colon) and rectum

In the large intestine, or colon, salts and water are absorbed from the liquefied food, leaving a semi-solid residue called feces (stool). Peristalsis moves the stool from the right side of your lower abdomen (where the colon begins) over to the left side of your lower abdomen, where the colon prepares for evacuation through the rectum. When food enters your stomach, an automatic reflex—called the *gastrocolic reflex*—sends nerve impulses into the smooth muscles of the colon, causing contractions to begin. This reflex is responsible for a baby's need to pass a bowel movement either during or shortly after drinking milk. The larger the meal and the higher the fat content, the stronger the gastrocolic reflex. In some patients with IBS, the gastrocolic reflex is overactive and causes abnormal cramping and diarrhea after eating.

When the stool enters the rectum, stretching causes the muscles of the lower rectum and anus to relax so that the stool can be eliminated by defecation. The internal and external anal sphincters are located at the end of the rectum. These sphincters serve as gatekeepers that prevent unwanted passage of the stool and permit purposeful defecation.

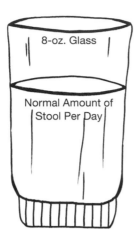

The normal bowel pattern for people in the United States ranges from three bowel movements per day to three per week. The normal amount of stool passed in a 24-hour period would not quite fill an 8-ounce glass.

Now that you have reviewed the anatomy and physiology of the gut, you are prepared to take your next lesson on the Mind/Brain-Gut Connection, where you will discover the "causes" of IBS.

# Chapter 11

## *The Causes of IBS*

A steady stream of messages flows back and
forth between the brain and the gut.
— *The Second Brain: The Scientific
Basis of Gut Instinct*
Michael D. Gershon, M.D.
Columbia University

A good set of bowels is worth more to
a man than any quantity of brains.
— Josh Billings
19th Century Humorist

The big brain in your head is connected to a "little-brain-in-the-gut" called the enteric nervous system, or ENS. The central nervous system (CNS) and the ENS are connected and communication is bi-directional, or two-way. This is the Mind/Brain-Gut Connection, which is a subcomponent of the three MindBodySpirit communication systems. Both brains act independently and interdependently. When homeostasis and the Mind/Brain-Gut Connection are disturbed by allostatic load and the bad stress response, functional gut symptoms, including those leading to the diagnosis of IBS, are generated. You will need to think differently (systematically rather than linearly) to understand the cause of IBS. Your symptoms are not imagined and all in your head. They are in your mind, brain, body and spirit!

Do you remember . . .

- That funny feeling in your stomach when you first fell in love?
- The butterflies in your stomach before the big game?
- The nausea and gastrointestinal upset you suffered before giving that speech?
- The cramps and diarrhea you got before a big job interview?

Most people know intuitively and by experience that there is a Mind/Brain-Gut Connection. Scientific studies show that most people experience unpleasant gut symptoms associated with stressors/triggers.

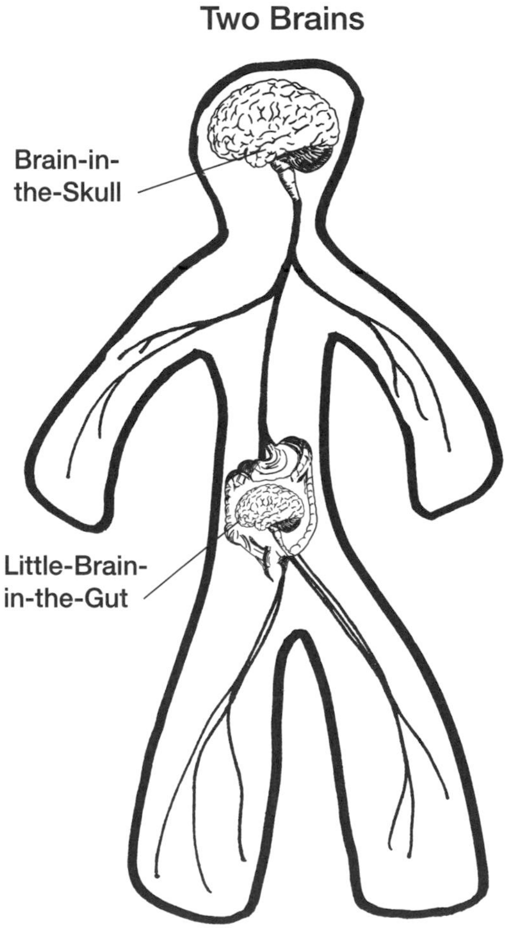

**Two Brains**

Brain-in-the-Skull

Little-Brain-in-the-Gut

Figure 11.1

# The Little-Brain-in-the-Gut (ENS)

There are two "brains" in your body. One brain is within your skull and is part of the central nervous system, or CNS. But you probably never realized that you have a second brain in the lining of your esophagus, stomach, small intestine, colon and rectum called the enteric nervous system, or ENS. Dr. Jack Wood, a physiologist at The Ohio State University and a pioneer in gut research, calls the ENS "the little-brain-in-the-gut" (Figure 11.1).

The CNS and the ENS closely resemble one another, because they both develop from the same embryonic tissue. Later, they take different developmental paths, but they continue to have similar nerve tissue and neurochemical communication receptor sites. All of the neurochemicals in the CNS are also found in the ENS.

Dr. Wood found that the ENS contains its own programs (much like computer programs) that are designed to protect you. These programs respond to perceived threats to homeostasis (triggers/stressors) in the same way that the limbic system (emotional motor system) of the central nervous system responds (Step 2). Dr. Wood has described several programs. For example, one is the "Power Propulsion (Anal Direction)" program that is designed to move digestive contents out through the rectum and anus. Stressors/triggers that activate this program, such as gastrointestinal infections, stimulate cramping and diarrhea to move the threat (infection) out of your gut. 💻Learn more about "the-little-brain-in-the-gut."

# Mind/Brain-Gut Connection

The big brain in your head and the little-brain-in-your-gut mutually influence one another. Gut sensations originating from the circuitry of nerves in the wall of the gut travel up the spinal cord and finally reach the brain. Transmission is bi-directional; it is a two-way street. The gut affects the brain, and the brain affects the gut. The responses (your symptoms, or "gut feelings") of the ENS to various environmental triggers/stressors are often reflected in the CNS, and vice versa. As we said, many healthy people experience diarrhea and other digestive symptoms when exposed to various stressors. In addition, many depressed patients suffer from altered bowel habits, such as diarrhea or constipation. In this way, perceived stress and psychological pain trigger or aggravate gut symptoms. In turn, gut symptoms may cause emotional stress and psychological unrest.

# Causes of Functional Gut Symptoms and IBS

Emeran A. Mayer, M.D., Chair of the University of California Los Angeles (UCLA) Mind-Body Collaborative Research Center and Head of the UCLA/CURE Neuroenteric Disease Program, Division of Digestive Diseases, has described an emerging disease model for IBS and functional gut syndromes. It is the response to stressors/triggers by the emotional motor system (limbic system) of the central nervous system that accounts for the symptoms of IBS (*American Journal of Medicine,* 1999 November 8;107(5A):12S–19S). This response of the emotional motor system may or may not be associated with the conscious experience of feelings of fear or anxiety. 🖳Learn more about <u>Dr. Mayer's disease model of IBS</u>.

Douglas A. Drossman, M.D., Co-Director of the University of North Carolina Center for Functional GI & Motility Disorders, says that IBS can be understood as a disorder of brain-gut regulation and that the symptoms derive from a dysregulation (disturbance) of the two-way communication between the gut and the brain (*Annual Reviews of Medicine,* 2001;52: 319–38). He emphasizes that the biopsychosocial model described in Chapter 4 integrates the physical, psychological and social factors that contribute to the symptom experience. 🖳 Learn more about <u>Dr. Drossman's biopsychosocial model of IBS</u>.

In Chapter 9, you learned how allostatic load and the bad stress response disturb homeostasis and the MindBodySpirit Connection, which results in functional symptoms leading to diagnosis of functional syndromes. Figure 11.2, "Causes of IBS," focuses upon the imbalance and disturbance of the Mind/Brain-Gut Connection, which is a subcomponent of the MindBodySpirit communication systems. Note that it is based upon the "MindBodySpirit Model of Bad Stress Response" depicted in Figure 9.2 from Chapter 9.

There are four main causes of functional gut symptoms that led to your diagnosis of IBS.

## 1.  Gut reactions to stressors/triggers

People normally respond to certain triggers (such as gut infections and fatty foods) with gut symptoms (such as abdominal cramping and diarrhea) through the good stress response that was described in Chapter 8. But those with IBS are more susceptible and sensitive to stressors/triggers because of the disturbed Mind/Brain-Gut Connection.

# MindBodySpirit Model of Causes of IBS

MindBodySpirit Modifying Factors: Spirituality, Faith and Hope; Sharing and Expressing Your Feelings; Changing the Meaning of an Event (Changing Your Thoughts, Feelings, Attitudes or Beliefs); Healthy Lifestyle Choices and Behavior; Medication and Other Treatments

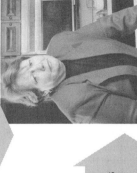

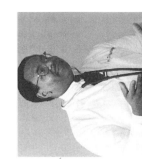

Symptoms and Disease

Doctor/Patient Relationship, Diagnosis, Education, Treatment

Psychological Distress

Neuromatrix

"Bad Stress" Response and Disturbed MindBodySpirit Connection

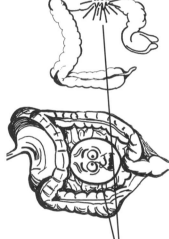

Spasm

Sensitivity

Perceived Threat to Homeostasis

Genetics and Early Life Experiences

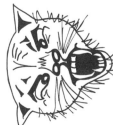

Stressors/ Triggers

Symptom Expression Through MindBodySpirit Communication Systems

Figure 11.2

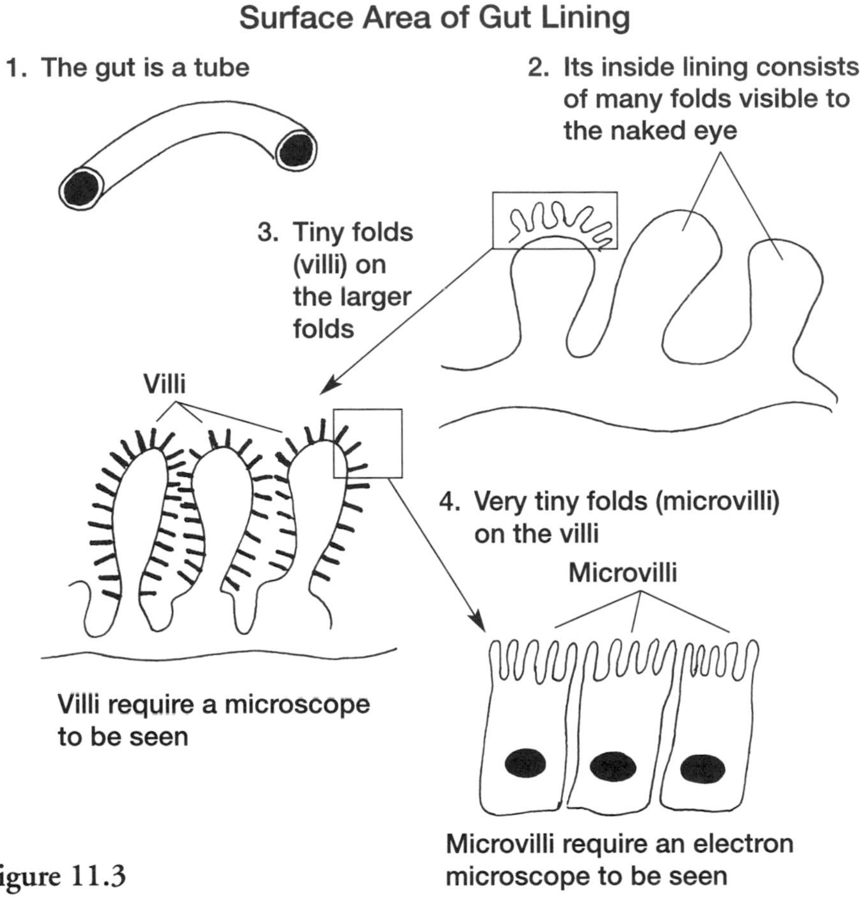

## Surface Area of Gut Lining

**1. The gut is a tube**

**2. Its inside lining consists of many folds visible to the naked eye**

**3. Tiny folds (villi) on the larger folds**

Villi

**4. Very tiny folds (microvilli) on the villi**

Microvilli

**Villi require a microscope to be seen**

**Figure 11.3**

**Microvilli require an electron microscope to be seen**

Your senses are involved in the detection and perception of stressors/triggers. You are familiar with the five senses—taste, smell, sight, hearing and touch. Your skin is the main body surface that is "in touch" with the world around you. Its surface area is about 2 square yards. By contrast, the surface area of the lining of your gut is about 5,250 square yards—the size of a football field (Figure 11.3).

So, the gut is an internal sensory system that interfaces with both the environment and the MindBodySpirit communication systems. UCLA gastroenterologist Emeran Mayer, M.D., says, ". . . most people generally think about events in the world around us, interfacing with our special senses and our external surface. However . . . our interactions with the world are much more extensive and intimate when we include in this interaction

our internal surface—the lining of the digestive system"
(*The Neurobiology Basis of Mind Body Medicine,* International Foundation for Functional Gastrointestinal Disorders, 2000). Food intake—which actually is the ingestion of bites of your external environment—can be a trigger/stressor of the internal sensory system of your gut.

Internal Gut
Trigger/Stressor

Much of what happens in the process of triggering the bad stress response occurs unconsciously. But both conscious awareness of what is happening to your gut and either elimination or reduction of identified triggers are important strategies for healing. In addition to those triggers you already learned about in Chapter 8, certain internal stressors/triggers deserve special mention with regard to your IBS. They are listed in Table 11.1. Some of these triggers will be addressed later in the book. One deserves special emphasis here: inflammation and infection.

---

Table 11.1

## Internal Gut Triggers/Stressors

| | |
|---|---|
| Foods | Hormones (e.g., menstrual cycle, menopause) |
| Dietary substances (e.g., sorbitol) | |
| Caffeine | Seasonal changes |
| Infection and inflammation | Perceived stress and psycho-social problems |
| Alcohol | |
| Drugs and medications | Poisons and toxins |

*Infection and inflammation.*   An infection of the gut is an important internal trigger/stressor that can mark the onset of IBS. A recent scientific study confirms previous studies as well as the clinical experience of gastroenterologists: about a quarter to a third of patients with diarrhea-predominant IBS report a previous history of an acute gastroenteritis. Risk factors for developing this "post-infectious IBS" include female sex, anxiety, depression, having other chronic functional symptoms and/or syndromes and adverse stressful life experiences in the previous year (*Gut,* 1999;44:400–406). Furthermore, the longer the initial illness, the more likely it was that IBS developed. For example, the risk was more than ten times greater if the initial diarrhea lasted for more than 21 days compared with diarrhea lasting less than seven days.

You have learned that medical tests, such as biopsies of the digestive tract, are normal in people with IBS. But some patients with post-infectious IBS do have colon biopsies that show an increase of what are called chronic inflammatory cells when viewed through a microscope, even though the appearance of the bowel is normal when viewed through a colonoscope (*Gut,* 2000;47:804–811). The evidence is accumulating that the bad stress response discussed in Chapter 9 can increase susceptibility to the development of IBS following exposure to the "threat" of an infectious internal stressor/trigger. Furthermore, the bad stress response may persist as a result of the triggering infection.

## 2.  Altered gut motility and spasm

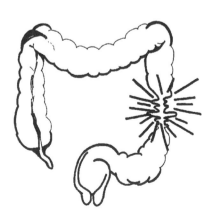

Disturbance in the Mind/Brain-Gut Connection leads to faulty regulation of gut motility and peristalsis, which can also result in spasm. These effects are largely mediated through the autonomic nervous system, which is one of the three MindBodySpirit communication systems described in Chapter 7. Disturbances in motility are responsible for IBS symptoms—abdominal pain, diarrhea, constipation or any combination of them. However, research has shown that some of the same motility disturbances that occur with IBS can also occur in healthy people.

Furthermore, IBS symptoms are not always accompanied by motility abnormalities, and motility abnormalities are not always accompanied by symptoms. There is another reason for the discomfort and pain of IBS—increased gut sensitivity.

## 3.  Increased gut sensitivity

Research has conclusively shown that patients with IBS have enhanced sensation and perception of what is happening in their digestive tract. They can feel things in their throat, chest, abdomen and rectum that other people cannot feel. What they feel can be uncomfortable and even painful. Doctors call this *enhanced visceral nociception.* Another way of looking at this is that the internal pain threshold for patients with IBS and other functional GI disorders is reduced. Even the sensation of normal peristaltic activity, movement and distention of the gut by food and gas may be experienced as uncomfortable. Alterations in the pain and symptom modulation subsystems of the MindBodySpirit communication systems are responsible (Chapter 7).

## 4.  Psychological distress

Allostatic load and the bad stress response are responsible for increased symptom vigilance. This means that you are more likely to pay attention to symptoms and be concerned by them. Furthermore, scientific studies have confirmed a common association of anxiety and depression with IBS and other functional diagnoses. Anxiety and depression are not the direct cause of IBS and other functional symptoms and syndromes, but there is emerging scientific evidence that anxiety and depression may be generated by the same processes that lead to functional symptoms and syndromes: allostatic load and the bad stress response. Associated anxiety and/or depression can amplify and worsen symptoms.

## System Thinking

You can appreciate now that there is no single cause of IBS. You will need to think about your symptoms and diagnosis differently. Look at Figure 11.4.

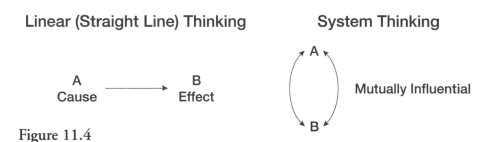

**Figure 11.4**

With linear or straight-line thinking, you assume that things are influenced only in one direction: A causes B. But system thinking allows you to think in terms of loops instead of straight lines. Both A and B influence one another and each is influenced by the other. So, understanding the cause of IBS and other functional gut syndromes requires a system appreciation of both the MindBodySpirit and the Mind/Brain-Gut Connection and their interrelatedness with genetics and the environment.

Your symptoms are not imagined or all in your head. They are in your mind, brain, body and spirit!

In the next chapter, you will learn more about gut feelings and the emotional brain.

# Chapter 12

## *The Emotional Brain and Gut*

The English language is full of expressions that suggest a long history
of implicit understanding amongst its users of the important role of the
viscera, in particular the digestive tract and cardiovascular systems, in
the emotional and cognitive functions of the brain.
– Emeran Mayer, M.D., Gastroenterologist
Director, UCLA/CURE Neuroenteric Disease Program

---

Do these phrases sound familiar to you? *There is a lump in my throat.
You make me sick to my stomach. I have butterflies (in my stomach).
You nauseate me.* These sayings all indicate that there is a well-under-
stood relationship between emotions, such as anger and fear, and unpleasant gut sensations and feelings. Furthermore, the saying, *I have
a gut feeling about this,* implies an understanding of an inner intelligence that is based upon prior experiences. Emotional gut responses
are not necessarily associated with conscious feeling of emotion. The
emotions are embodied and you can learn from them.

---

## Gut Feelings

Common expressions like, "I have a gut feeling about this," or "My gut
instinct tells me," refer to what Daniel Goleman calls emotional intelligence (in his book, *Emotional Intelligence*). Gut feelings refer to a type of
inner intelligence that seems to be based upon prior experiences. Antonio
Damasio, M.D., author of the book *Descartes' Error: Emotion, Reason,
and the Human Brain* and *The Feeling of What Happens: Body and Emotion in the Making of Consciousness,* says that gut feelings are based upon
previous life experience that was also associated with a gut sensation. He
proposes that part or most of our rational decision-making may be based

upon the imprinted emotional content of prior experience. In other words, that gut feeling is reminding you of something!

# The Neurobiology of Emotion

The neurobiology of emotions is a relatively new field of study. A pioneer in this area is Joseph LeDoux, Ph.D., professor at the Center for Neural Science at New York University and author of the book *The Emotional Brain: The Mysterious Underpinnings of Emotional Life.* Some of his important discoveries are relevant to IBS and other functional symptoms. Let's look at these in more detail.

### Emotions: Designed to protect and teach

Remember the tiger in your path? Whether it is physically there or only in your mind, the stress response that is triggered is very real. Generated by the emotional brain and communicated through the MindBodySpirit communication systems, this emotional good stress (fight-or-flight) response is built into you—and into all animals—for protection.

In his book *Why Zebras Don't Get Ulcers,* Stanford neuroscientist Robert Sapolsky says that if you were a zebra and were threatened by a tiger, your digestive processes would not be important. Blood flow would be shifted away from the gut to the muscles (so you could run away), and you might vomit and have diarrhea so that you would be lighter and able to run faster.

You also learn through emotional experiences. When you have a life experience that is accompanied by a gut feeling, that feeling will be remembered. If you have a similar experience in the future, then that gut feeling will be integrated with your thoughts to help you make a decision. Your gut feelings represent part of your built-in capacity for intuition. Gut feelings help the zebra remember not only the tiger but also assist it in responding appropriately to any similarly threatening animal.

### Gut responses: Not necessarily conscious

All animals, including humans, must be able to detect and react to danger. Dr. LeDoux emphasizes, "It is possible for emotions to be triggered in us without the cortex knowing exactly what is going on." Thus, if a stressor/trigger is perceived by the MindBodySpirit Connection to be a threat to homeostasis, then the MindBodySpirit communication systems generate an emotional stress response that can lead to bodily symptoms such as those described in this chapter and throughout this book. Symptoms that result from danger and threat—such as nausea, vomiting and diarrhea—affect you whether you are conscious of the actual stressor/trigger or not. Furthermore, if you were to take a psychological test, it might not indicate that you have any problem with anxiety or fear. This really is a "crouching tiger in the mind"!

## Emotions and feelings are not the same

From a neurobiological standpoint, emotions are generated in your body when your limbic system (emotional motor system) generates nerve cell firings and chemical release. When—and if—your mind becomes consciously aware of these bodily emotions, they are called *feelings*. Dr. LeDoux says, "We come into the world capable of being afraid and capable of being happy, but we must learn which things make us afraid and which make us happy." Your good stress fight-or-flight response generates emotional reactions (sensations) in your body that are designed to protect you, whether your mind is aware of these bodily emotions or not. If you also become aware that you are afraid or anxious, then bodily emotions become mental feelings. Feelings are emotional responses (sensations) in the body that are consciously perceived in the mind.

The distinction between emotions and feelings is the basis for many forms of bodywork that involve releasing bodily emotions of which you have no conscious awareness. One of us (Neil) once had a deep massage in his neck area and began to spontaneously cry, as if some "sadness" was being released from his muscles. He had no awareness of being sad, but it felt good to release the emotions and the massage felt good too! Many times, you may find yourself clenching your fist or grinding your teeth, unaware that you are doing it. These actions reflect emotional stress in your body, even though you may not feel stressed or anxious. These represent your body emotions—in other words, times when your body is feeling your feelings without your conscious awareness!

# The Emotional Connection

Robert and Lydia Dorsky (Healthcare Communications, Short Hills, N.J.) produce educational materials on health and medicine. In their article entitled "The Mind-Gut Connection" (*Digestive Health & Nutrition,* May/June 2000) they wrote, "When you suffer from stomach problems, your emotions may play an important role in your digestive system's workings. Gastroenterologists have found that, for many patients, treatment for some digestive disorders must be geared toward the emotional as well as the physical aspects of their condition." In the same article, Ray Clouse, M.D., from Washington University School of Medicine in St. Louis says, "It is unacceptable to simply say that your bowel problem is making you depressed, and so we should just ignore the depression until the bowel problem is fixed. There is often an interaction between emotions, the brain, and the bowels, and this means treating the entire problem, not just the gut."

"The emotions are embodied," writes Ian R. McWhinney, M.D., preeminent Canadian family medicine specialist and author of *A Textbook of Family Medicine* (*Annals of Internal Medicine,* 1997).

Now that you know how emotional stress responses can affect your body, mind and spirit, you are ready to review the symptoms of IBS and other common functional gut syndromes in the next chapter.

# Chapter 13

## *Symptoms of IBS and Other Functional Gut Syndromes*

**Man should strive to have his intestines relaxed all the days of his life.**
– Moses Maimonides
12th century healer and physician

> The functional colonic symptoms that lead to the diagnosis of IBS are chronic or recurrent abdominal discomfort or pain, particularly in the lower abdominal area, that is related to a change in stool frequency or consistency. Typically, having a bowel movement relieves the pain or discomfort. Many functional gut symptoms lead to the diagnosis of one or more functional gut disorders, or syndromes. These disorders are defined by the symptom-based ROME II diagnostic criteria.

## Normal Bowel Function

The normal bowel pattern for people in the United States ranges from three bowel movements per day to three bowel movements per week. The normal amount of stool passed in a 24-hour period would not quite fill an 8-ounce glass. Stool form can be quite variable, and gastroenterologists have actually classified various stool forms into seven types (Table 13.1).

## The Symptoms of IBS

Research has shown that the symptoms of IBS are found in up to twenty percent of people in the United States. Less than one-half of people who

| Table 13.1 | |
| :-- | :-- |
| **The Bristol (England) Stool Form Scale*** | |
| **Type** | **Description of Stool** |
| 1 | Separate hard lumps like nuts (difficult to pass) |
| 2 | Sausage shaped but lumpy |
| 3 | Like a sausage but with cracks on its surface |
| 4 | Like a sausage or snake, smooth and soft |
| 5 | Soft blobs with clear-cut edges (passed easily) |
| 6 | Fluffy pieces with raged edges, a mushy stool |
| 7 | Watery, no solid pieces, *entirely liquid* |

*\* British Medical Journal, 1990;300:439–40.*

have these symptoms consult a doctor for them. IBS symptoms, which are related to the colon, include abdominal pain or discomfort associated with disturbance of bowel function—diarrhea, constipation or alternation between diarrhea and constipation.

Table 13.2 lists the symptoms that doctors recognize as typical of IBS. ROME II criteria are symptom-based diagnostic criteria for functional gut syndromes developed by an international consensus of experts. Information on the ROME II Criteria is available on the Internet at www.romecriteria.org.

Other symptoms of IBS may include:

- Abnormal bowel frequency (more than three per day or less than three per week)
- Abnormal stool form (lumpy/hard or loose/watery stool)
- Abnormal stool passage, such as straining, urgency or the feeling that you have not completely emptied your rectum after a bowel movement
- Passage of mucus in or on the stool
- Abdominal bloating, distention or swelling.

---

Table 13.2

### Symptoms of Irritable Bowel Syndrome (IBS)*
### (Affects one in every five people in the United States)

If you have experienced abdominal discomfort or pain for at least 12 weeks (not necessarily consecutive weeks) in the last year, and if your discomfort or pain is accompanied by two or more of the following features, then you may have IBS:

- Your pain or discomfort is relieved after you have a bowel movement
- When your pain starts, you have a change in your usual number of bowel movements (either more or fewer)
- When your pain or discomfort starts, you have either softer or harder stools than usual.

* Based upon ROME II Criteria. Adapted from the American Digestive Health Foundation *IBS Consumer Brochure,* which is based upon Thompson, W.G., et. al., "Functional bowel disorders and functional abdominal pain." *Gut* Vol. 45 Supplement II, 43–47, 1999. This brochure may be viewed on the Internet at www.gastro.org/adhf

# Abdominal Pain and Cramping

The abdominal pain and discomfort associated with IBS are usually located in the lower abdomen below the belly button. Most commonly, the pain occurs in your lower left side, but the pain can actually occur anywhere in the abdomen. The pain can be dull, sharp, cramping or constant. Typically, but not always, it can be relieved by having a bowel movement or passing flatus (gas). Often, people notice that they have more frequent or looser bowel movements when they are having trouble with the pain. Others notice the pain more when they are constipated. Some note that pain is worsened with defecation.

The pain can be referred into other bodily locations, which can be a source of confusion for patients and doctors. Common referral areas are the chest, pelvis or legs. It may help to further elaborate on the symptoms of IBS.

### Attacks of severe abdominal pain

Some people with IBS have sudden attacks of abdominal pain that can be so severe that they visit a doctor immediately or go to the emergency room. IBS is a common cause of brief hospital admissions for observation and evaluation of abdominal pain.

### Hyperactive gastrocolic reflex

Many people with IBS have the urgent need to have a bowel movement soon after eating, which is a phenomenon called hyperactive gastrocolic reflex. This can be such a big problem that many people will not eat for the entire day, waiting until they get home at night so they can work without the embarrassment of the urgent need to use the bathroom.

### Morning rush

A common symptom pattern is the occurrence of diarrhea and/or stool urgency in the morning. This can happen either immediately upon awakening from sleep or be triggered by eating breakfast. Some people have difficulty getting to work on time because of this "morning rush."

### Urgency to have a bowel movement

The urge to have a bowel movement can be very sudden and unpredictable, or it can be associated with certain situations, like going out to eat or to the grocery. People may avoid these situations or resolve to never go anywhere without knowing exactly where the bathroom is.

## Severity and Impact

The severity of the symptoms of IBS varies from mild and annoying to severe and disabling, and its impact varies from person to person. IBS can cause enough discomfort that daily activities are altered and performance of ordinary activities is impaired. For example, IBS is a one of the most common reasons for missing work. Patients with IBS have an average of 13 days per year absent from work, while the rest of the population has 5 days per year (*Digestive Diseases and Sciences,* 1993;38:1569–1580).

The economic impact of functional gut syndromes is remarkable. The annual direct (health care expenditures) and indirect (loss of work productivity) costs have been estimated at $41 billion in eight major industrialized countries, including $26 billion in the United States and $4 billion each in Japan and Germany (*European Journal of Surgery,* 1998;582: 62–64).

# IBS Symptom Patterns

Doctors try to determine the patient's predominant symptom pattern, because this can be helpful in designing a treatment plan. The most common symptom patterns are referred to as A-IBS, D-IBS and C-IBS.

## Alternating IBS (A-IBS)

This is the most common IBS symptom pattern, which is present in about 50 percent of cases. The bowel pattern is irregular and alternates between diarrhea and constipation. For example, there may be no bowel movements for several days and then diarrhea throughout a day. Stool character and consistency may be very erratic: thin pencil-like and ribbon-like stool may occur intermittently as spasm in the sigmoid colon narrows and molds the stool diameter (Figure 13.1). This can also cause the stool to look like the pellets that rabbits pass—what doctors call "scybalous" stools.

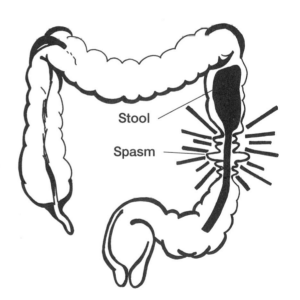

Stool

Spasm

**Figure 13.1**

## Diarrhea-predominant IBS (D-IBS)

In this symptom pattern, diarrhea predominates. Patients report more than three bowel movements per day, loose or watery stools and an urgency to have a bowel movement. Approximately thirty percent of IBS patients have this pattern.

Another functional gastrointestinal disorder in which diarrhea is the predominant symptom is chronic functional diarrhea. ROME II criteria for this syndrome include at least 12 weeks, which need not be consecutive, in the preceding 12 months of loose (mushy) or watery stools that are present over ¾ of the time *without abdominal pain.*

## Constipation-predominant IBS (C-IBS)

In this symptom pattern, constipation predominates. Patients report infrequent bowel movements, hard or lumpy stools, a sensation of incomplete rectal evacuation and excessive straining. Approximately 20 percent of IBS patients have this pattern.

The definition of constipation as having fewer than 3 bowel movements per week is based upon epidemiological studies of large numbers of people. However, many who report that they have constipation have bowel movements on a daily basis while complaining of straining during defecation or of being unable to completely empty the rectum.

Another functional gastrointestinal disorder in which constipation predominates is chronic functional constipation. ROME II criteria for functional constipation include at least 12 weeks, which need not be consecutive, in the preceding 12 months of two or more of: (1) straining with over one-fourth of defecations, (2) lumpy or hard stools with over one-fourth of defecations, (3) sensation of incomplete evacuation of the rectum with over one-fourth of defecations, (4) sensation of obstruction/blockage of the anus or rectum with over one-fourth of defecations, (5) use of manual maneuvers to facilitate over one-fourth of defecations (e.g., using fingers around or in the rectum or vagina to help get the stool out of the rectum) and/or (6) less than three defecations per week.

There are two points to stress regarding the criteria for chronic functional constipation. First, having fewer than 3 bowel movements per week alone is not sufficient for the diagnosis. It is necessary to have at least one other problem. Second, it is possible to have chronic functional constipation and three or more bowel movements per week.

# Other Functional Symptoms and Syndromes

In Chapters 1 and 2, you were introduced to the many functional gastro-intestinal symptoms and syndromes that may or may not be associated with IBS. The more common ones are described briefly here. 💻 Learn more about <u>functional gut symptoms and syndromes</u>.

For the most part, ROME II diagnostic criteria specify that the functional gut syndrome be present for at least 12 weeks, which need not be consecutive, in the preceding 12 months. The purpose for this is to separate these chronic conditions from transient and temporary gut symptoms, such as may occur with emotional distress or infection. The exception is functional abdominal pain syndrome (FAPS), in which the diagnostic criteria must have been present for at least six months. The functional gut diagnoses are based upon the absence of a structural or biochemical disorder or disease process. It is very common for functional gut symptoms and syndromes to overlap and occur together or with other functional bodily symptoms and syndromes. They also tend to come and go, change from one to another and fluctuate in severity.

## Globus

Studies show that, from time to time, most people experience a lump, foreign body sensation or sense of a ball in the throat when they have an intense emotional experience. The term *globus* is Latin for ball or globe. Functional globus is typically felt in the throat at the level of the Adam's apple. Globus must be distinguished from the medical problem called *dysphagia,* which occurs during eating and drinking. Dysphagia is a sensation of having actual difficulty with the act of swallowing or with movement of food or fluid through the esophagus. Food may actually stop on the way down. Dysphagia usually indicates an important problem that requires medical investigation. Unlike dysphagia, globus occurs between meals and is relieved by swallowing something.

## Functional abdominal bloating and distention

Functional abdominal bloating is described as a feeling of excessive abdominal pressure that may or may not be accompanied by actual visible abdominal distention or enlargement. Abdominal bloating can be uncomfortable and even painful. Furthermore, when associated with abdominal distention, bloating can make dressing awkward and contribute to poor self-image. Finally, bloating may induce an urge to pass gas that can be inconvenient or embarrassing and associated with anxiety. Bloating is seen more commonly in women than in men and tends to become more prominent towards the end of the day and in the pre-menstrual period.

Abdominal bloating may be part of IBS if the symptom is associated with abdominal pain and alterations in bowel habits. Bloating may also be associated with functional dyspepsia (see following discussion), making the symptom difficult to differentiate from the fullness that occurs following meals. Bloating may also be associated with gas.

## Functional dyspepsia

The term *dyspepsia* refers to pain or discomfort centered in the upper abdomen. "Centered" means that the symptom is located in or around the midline. Pain that is located in either the right upper quadrant or the left upper quadrant is not considered to be dyspepsia. Dyspepsia may or may not be associated with meals. A common disease cause of dyspepsia is peptic ulcer of the stomach or duodenum.

By definition, functional dyspepsia is not caused by a disease process, such as ulcer. Furthermore, it is not IBS, meaning that the symptom is not exclusively relieved by defecation or associated with the onset of a change in stool frequency or stool form. Nevertheless, functional dyspepsia and IBS often coexist.

## Functional nausea and vomiting

Nausea is usually described as a queasy, sick to the stomach sensation that may progress to the feeling of impending vomiting and ultimately to vomiting. Chronic nausea is a common functional symptom, while functional vomiting is rare. Interestingly, ROME II diagnostic criteria have been developed for functional vomiting but not for functional nausea. Some patients with chronic nausea describe an associated upper abdominal discomfort that could be considered to be dyspepsia (see preceding discussion), so chronic nausea is usually considered to be a form of chronic dyspepsia. Associated symptoms related to the autonomic nervous system are common, such as sweating and light-headedness. Finally, many report associated fatigue and even depression of mood.

## Excessive gas

Excessive gas can refer to one of four different symptoms. First, some patients refer to abdominal pain or discomfort as "gas." This may require medical investigation.

The second symptom is aerophagia, which refers to a repetitive pattern of swallowing or ingesting air that results in belching. Patients with aerophagia may belch to relieve abdominal discomfort. The air swallowing is usually an unconscious process that is unrelated to eating. Most of the time, chronic troublesome and repetitive aerophagia resulting in belching is diagnosed as functional aerophagia.

Third, gas may refer to perceived excessive rectal gas or flatulence (farting). Everyone produces gas and everyone passes it rectally. The amount of intestinal gas varies from individual to individual, and there is a wide range of what is considered normal. Scientific studies show that it is normal to pass up to 20 farts per day, so it is important to determine whether the number of farts passed per day is greater than 20. Flatulence may or may not have a bad smell. Flatulence occurs when indigestible carbohydrates pass into the colon, where they cannot be absorbed. Bacterial fermentation of these carbohydrates produces gas. Treatment of flatulence is primarily dietary (Chapter 17), but may also include medication or natural remedies (Chapter 18).

Fourth, some patients consider functional bloating and distention to be a gas problem. Bloating and gas problems with belching and/or flatulence may or may not coexist. Some who suffer with bloating complain of difficulty passing gas orally or rectally. Bloating is a common symptom in those who have a problem with excessive belching. By contrast, many who complain of excessive flatulence do not report bloating.

## Functional heartburn

Heartburn is defined as an episodic burning sensation behind the breastbone related to gastroesophageal reflux disease (GERD). GERD affects 20 to 30 percent of people in the United States and is related to the reflux or return of stomach acid into the esophagus. Yet, gastroenterologists commonly see patients describe heartburn that either fails to respond or responds incompletely to strong antisecretory drugs called proton pump inhibitors (such as Prilosec, Prevacid, Aciphex, Protonix and Nexium). This is functional heartburn. It is important to recognize functional heartburn to avoid unnecessary surgery from a misdiagnosis of GERD.

## Functional chest pain of presumed esophageal origin

If chest pain is not related to an abnormality of the heart (angina) or lungs, or to chest wall musculoskeletal strain or inflammation, then it is usually attributed to the esophagus. Between 15 percent and 30 percent of coronary angiograms performed for the evaluation of chest pain are normal. The most common cause of esophageal chest pain is GERD (see preceding discussion). However, a sensitive and spastic esophagus may be unrelated to GERD. This is functional chest pain of presumed esophageal origin, which occurs in the middle of the chest. It is important to stress that functional chest pain can be confused with cardiac angina or pain related to other esophageal disorders, including gastroesophageal reflux disease (GERD) and a rare condition called achalasia. Thus, it is necessary to consider these disorders before the diagnosis of functional chest pain of presumed esophageal origin is established.

## Functional gallbladder and biliary pain

Gallbladder and biliary (bile duct) pain is usually described as severe steady pain that is located in the middle upper abdomen above the belly button (the epigastrium) and/or in the right upper quadrant. It lasts for 30 minutes or more, with pain-free intervals that can last for days, weeks and months. Gallstones are usually responsible, but some patients have gallbladder or biliary pain that is not gallstone associated. These conditions are called functional disorders of the biliary tract and pancreas.

## Functional abdominal pain syndrome (FAPS)

Functional abdominal pain syndrome (FAPS), also called "chronic idiopathic abdominal pain," or "chronic functional abdominal pain," is continuous or nearly continuous abdominal pain that has been present for at least 6 months and which cannot be explained by medical testing. The pain is usually constant or frequently recurrent and tends to involve a large portion of the abdomen. The main difference between the less common FAPS and IBS is that there is either no or little association of the pain with bowel function. Furthermore, the pain is usually unrelated to eating or to menses.

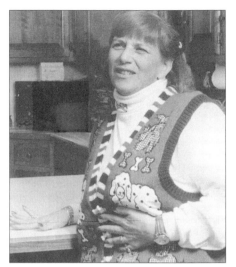

**Pain of FAPS Is Usually Unrelated to Bowel Function**

## Functional rectal pain

There are two functional rectal pain syndromes. The first and most common one is called proctalgia fugax. This is a sudden and often severe pain in the anus or lower rectum that lasts for several seconds to several minutes and then completely disappears. It is common for the symptom to awaken people from sleep, and it can occur after sexual activity. The attacks are usually infrequent.

The second is levator ani syndrome, which is chronic or recurrent rectal pain or aching that occurs episodically for 20 minutes or longer. The pain is often described as a dull ache or pressure sensation that is vague and felt high in the rectal area. It commonly seems worse with sitting than with standing or lying down. When the doctor examines the anus and rectum, the tenderness is most commonly noted more on the left than the right side.

## Bladder and gynecologic symptoms and syndromes

The bowel, pelvic organs and bladder can be associated with remarkably similar symptoms. Scientific studies confirm that women with IBS tend to suffer more painful menstrual periods, commonly report that their IBS symptoms are worse at the time of their menstrual periods and often have dyspareunia (pain with sexual intercourse). More than 50 percent of patients consulting a gynecologist for lower abdominal and/or pelvic pain diagnosed as chronic pelvic pain syndrome (see Chapter 2) have associated IBS.

The bladder symptoms that are most commonly associated with IBS are increased frequency in passing urine, urgency to urinate and sometimes urinary incontinence. This in turn can result in mistaken diagnosis of recurrent cystitis (bladder infection) with repeated antibiotic treatment. Furthermore, a urologist may diagnose interstitial cystitis, or irritable bladder syndrome (see Chapter 2).

In the medical journal *Practical Gastroenterology* (April, 2000), Dr. Peter J. Whorwell, an English gastroenterologist, says that gynecological symptoms are most likely IBS related if the pain is associated with bowel function, involves the upper abdomen above the belly button and/or is associated with dyspepsia and/or nausea (see earlier discussion). So if surgery for an apparent gynecological or bladder problem is recommended, be sure that you and your doctor consider that at least some of the symptoms could be IBS-related and would not be expected to respond.

In the next chapter, you will learn how doctors diagnosis IBS.

# Chapter 14
## *The Diagnosis of IBS*

It is of the highest importance in the art of detection to recognize,
out of a number of facts, which are incidental and which are vital.
— Sherlock Holmes
as quoted by Sir Arthur Conan Doyle

---

This chapter will help you to understand how your doctor may go
about diagnosing your symptoms as consistent with IBS. The diagnosis of IBS is based upon: (1) the identification of certain symptoms
(positive symptom diagnosis), (2) determination of the predominant
symptom pattern (alternating diarrhea and constipation, mostly diarrhea or mostly constipation), (3) the absence of "red flags" that signal
the possibility of another disease masquerading as IBS, (4) identification of certain key historical features (history of abuse, persistent
symptoms following the acute onset of gastroenteritis and associated
anxiety or depression), (5) recognition of associated functional symptoms and syndromes, (6) clues in the family history, (7) consideration of differential diagnosis and (8) the judicious application of
appropriate medical testing.

---

## Positive Symptom Diagnosis

The evaluation of patients with suspected IBS can vary depending upon
symptoms, age and general health status. Until recently, IBS was a diagnosis of exclusion, which means that doctors often had to perform many tests
in order to exclude other possible diseases. However, doctors now attempt
to generate a positive symptom diagnosis. This means that they look for
symptoms and characteristics shown to indicate the likely presence of a
functional gut disorder/syndrome. These are called ROME II diagnostic

criteria, which were developed when a multinational group of doctors and other professionals met in Rome, Italy, to develop diagnostic criteria for these problems. They developed this symptom-based, diagnostic classification system by reviewing published research studies and by group consensus. The criteria developed are similar to classification systems used in rheumatology and psychiatry. The Rome II criteria for IBS were presented in Chapter 13. 🖳 Learn more about <u>the Rome II criteria</u>.

## Predominant Symptom Pattern

As the next step in diagnosis, doctors try to determine whether there is a predominant symptom pattern, since this can be helpful in designing a treatment plan. There are three predominant symptom patterns, which were discussed in Chapter 13: A-IBS (alternating diarrhea and constipation); D-IBS (diarrhea predominant); and C-IBS (constipation predominant).

## "Red Flags" of Masquerading Disorders

In addition to characteristic symptom patterns, doctors must evaluate your condition carefully to uncover "red flags" that could signal the presence of a disease or disorder that may masquerade as IBS. When red flags are present, your doctor will probably need to order specialized tests. The most common red flags are:

- If your symptoms began later in life, especially after the age of 50. Most people with functional GI symptoms have had them earlier in life. If you develop new symptoms after age 50, it is particularly important to check for other diseases and disorders that might require completely different treatment.
- If your symptoms steadily and progressively get worse.
- If you have a change in the pattern of your symptoms, or new symptoms develop after a long period of time without symptoms.
- If you are frequently awakened at night by your symptoms.  Functional GI symptoms do not usually awaken people from sleep.

- If your symptoms developed shortly after you have been on antibiotics.
- If you have a fever with your symptoms.
- If you have unexplained weight loss.
- If you have rectal bleeding.
- If you have fat in your stools (steatorrhea). Oil droplets in the commode can be a sign of abnormal fat in the stool.
- If you are dehydrated.
- If you have an abnormal blood test (like anemia) or abnormal findings on physical examination like a lump or mass in the abdomen.
- If you have a family history of colorectal cancer, inflammatory bowel disease or celiac sprue.

# Key Historical Information

There are three important historical features that are directly relevant to the diagnosis and management of IBS.

## History of abuse

In Chapter 9, you discovered that early life events could alter the responsiveness of the MindBodySpirit Connection to stressors/triggers and the ability to adapt through allostasis, which renders a person susceptible to the bad stress response throughout life. Research has confirmed that a history of emotional, physical or sexual abuse is a frequent finding in women with IBS, particularly if the symptoms are severe. This can be understood from the perspective of the MindBodySpirit Connection, since severe abuse is often accompanied by unconscious repression of these painful memories. These repressed memories lie hidden—like the crouching tiger—in the unconscious mind and body memory, where they exert an excessive allostatic load on the mind, body and spirit. It is important to identify this history, since professional counseling is often necessary for full healing. Refer back to Figures 9.2 and 11.2 for a visual representation of how early life experience, such as abuse, can predispose to IBS.

### Onset and persistence following gut infection

Some patients with IBS report that their symptoms began with an acute gut infection such as viral gastroenteritis or a bacterial infection. This was addressed in Chapter 11, since infection and inflammation are stressors/triggers. It is further discussed below in the section on Differential Diagnosis.

### Associated anxiety or depression

In Chapter 11, you learned that IBS and other functional syndromes are commonly associated with psychological distress, including anxiety and depression. This association is important, since anxiety and depression can increase symptoms and concern about them. Successful management of IBS includes identifying (Chapter 32) and addressing (Chapter 18) associated anxiety and depression.

## Associated Functional Symptoms and Syndromes

As you learned in the first two chapters, many patients with IBS suffer from other functional symptoms and syndromes, both of the gut and involving other bodily systems. In other words, functional symptoms and syndromes commonly overlap. Many people have an irritable body syndrome! It is common for symptoms to vary and change, and even for one syndrome to disappear while another one develops.

## Family History

Your family history is important, because it can provide the doctor with valuable clues about what might be wrong with you. First-degree relatives (parents, brothers, sisters and children) are family members in whom the doctor is most interested. New research has shown that IBS and other functional gut disorders tend to run in families. You have learned that genetics (heredity) and the social environment of family are interrelated with the MindBodySpirit Connection. This also helps to explain why other diseases and disorders tend to run in families, which may provide clues to your differential diagnosis discussed next.

# Differential Diagnosis

There are several different disorders and diseases that the doctor needs to consider in what is called "differential diagnosis." These are conditions that could be masquerading as IBS and that require proper diagnosis and treatment (Table 14.1). Five of these disorders are discussed here. Learn more about <u>IBS differential diagnosis</u>.

---

Table 14.1

## Differential Diagnosis of IBS

* Inflammatory bowel disease
* Colorectal cancer
  Diverticulosis
  Medications affecting bowel pattern (constipating or
    diarrhea-causing agents)
  Gastrointestinal infections
  Lactose intolerance
* Endocrine disorders and tumors (thyroid disorders most
    commonly)
  Microscopic colitis
  Collagenous colitis
  Chronic intestinal idiopathic pseudo obstruction (very rare)
  Bacterial overgrowth
  Antibiotic associated infection *(Clostridium difficile)*
* Malabsorption syndromes (especially celiac sprue)

---

* Family history may be important

## Inflammatory bowel disease (IBD)

Inflammatory bowel disease (IBD) is always accompanied by inflammation in the intestinal lining that can be visibly detected by x-ray or colonoscopy, but IBS is not associated with visible inflammation. Review Chapter 11 for a discussion of infection and inflammation associated with IBS.

*Two forms of IBD.*   Approximately one million Americans are afflicted with IBD and the cause remains unknown. There are two forms of IBD (sometimes called "colitis")—each with a classical triad of symptoms (which are not always present). Ulcerative colitis is characterized by diarrhea, rectal bleeding and abdominal cramping. Crohn's disease is characterized by diarrhea, weight loss and abdominal pain.

*Help in this book for patients with IBD.*   Even though IBD patients may require treatment for inflammation and potential complications, the stress response can activate or aggravate IBD. UCLA gastroenterologist Dr. Emeran Mayer has authored two important medical articles discussing the scientific evidence of this important observation (*Gut,* 2000; 46:595–596 and *Gut,* 2000;47:861–869). University of North Carolina gastroenterologist Douglas Drossman has recently discussed the importance of psychosocial factors in Crohn's disease (*Surgical Clinics of North America,* February, 2001). Furthermore, many patients with IBD also have IBS. Dr. E. Jan Irvine and other investigators at McMaster University School of Medicine, Hamilton, Ontario, have confirmed that acute or chronic inflammation of the gut (infection, gastroenteritis or that associated with IBD) can cause persistent gut motility disturbance (spasm) and sensitivity. You have learned that there is often a poor correlation between the degree of inflammation or disease and the presence and severity of symptoms. For example, some patients with IBD have moderate to severe symptoms despite mild to absent active inflammation. It is very important for IBD patients and their doctors to recognize this common association of IBS and IBD in order to avoid unnecessary IBD treatment. Furthermore, the lessons of this book may help to relieve symptoms and quiet inflammation.

## Colon polyps and colon cancer

Having IBS does not increase the risk of developing colon or rectal polyps or cancer. However, it is important to consider the diagnosis of colorectal polyps or cancer whenever there is rectal bleeding, a new change of bowel pattern that lasts for more than two to three weeks, unexplained weight loss, iron deficiency anemia or a family history of colorectal polyps or cancer (mainly first degree relatives: mother, father, brother, sister or children).

## Diverticulosis

Diverticulosis of the colon is a very common condition that occurs when small outpouchings, called *diverticula,* form in the colon wall. Diverticulosis becomes more common with age, and as many as 50 percent of Americans over the age of 60 have the condition. Most people with diverticulosis are unaware that they have it, unless they develop a complication of either inflammation (diverticulitis) or rectal bleeding. Since diverticulosis and IBS are both common conditions, it is common for them to occur together.

## Celiac sprue

Celiac sprue, or gluten-sensitive enteropathy, is discussed in Chapter 17. This disorder is caused by a specific sensitivity to the grain products wheat, barley, rye and oats. New research conducted at the University of Maryland (www.celiaccenter.org) shows that as many as one in every 150 people in the United States may have celiac sprue. Having a family member with the diagnosis increases the likelihood that you will have it, as does having diarrhea and/or iron deficiency anemia. A blood test is available to screen for the condition.

## Bacterial overgrowth

Bacterial overgrowth in the small intestine can cause symptoms that are similar to those of IBS. It should be considered in the differential diagnosis of patients who report abdominal bloating/distention, diarrhea and/or flatulence after meals. Most patients who have bacterial overgrowth have a disorder or disease of the small intestine, such as inflammatory bowel disease (Crohn's disease), a history of previous intestinal surgery or partial obstruction (blockage). But occasionally, bacterial overgrowth can mimic or worsen IBS, even though there is no structural or disease state present. Medical testing for bacterial overgrowth is available and the condition is treatable with antibiotics. Also refer to the discussion on "Probiotics" in Chapter 18.

*Yeast infection.*   Even though candida (monilia) is a yeast rather than bacterial infection, there is considerable "pseudoscience" and misinformation regarding gut infection with yeast. There is no scientific evidence that candida or yeast either causes or triggers IBS (*New England Journal of Medicine,* 1990;323:1717–1723). Furthermore, there is no scientific evidence of a systemic yeast syndrome that could account for functional symptoms and syndromes (*New England Journal of Medicine,* 1990;323: 1717 and 1990;323:1766).

# Medical Testing

Based upon the approach that has been outlined here, you and your doctor can decide what medical testing will be necessary. This may include blood tests, flexible sigmoidoscopy, colonoscopy, biopsies and x-rays.

In the next chapter, we will dispel common myths and misunderstandings about IBS.

# Chapter 15
## *Myths and Misunderstandings*

Beauty is truth, truth beauty—that is all
Ye know on earth, and all ye need to know
– *Ode on a Grecian Urn*
John Keats

> There are several myths and misunderstandings about IBS and other functional gut disorders that should be clarified and dispelled in order to clear the way for healing.

## "It's All in Your Head," or "It's Just Stress."

It is impossible to separate mind, body and spirit. You should now understand how your thoughts, beliefs, attitudes, emotions, feelings and stress response are transmitted throughout your entire being by way of the three MindBodySpirit Connection communication systems. So your symptoms are not all in your head. They are in your mind, brain, body and spirit!

## "The Symptoms Are Minor."

While it is true that many people have mild and inconvenient symptoms, there are others who are significantly disabled and incapacitated by the symptoms of IBS. Remember that IBS is the second leading cause of missed work in the United States and is responsible for innumerable doctor and emergency room visits. Many people with IBS lead restricted lives and are afraid to leave home without knowing where all of the bathrooms

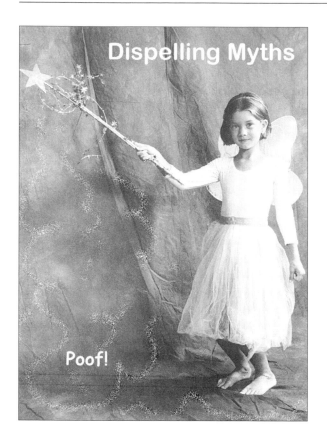

Dispelling Myths

Poof!

are located. IBS patients often completely avoid social activities. Relationships with family and co-workers may suffer.

## "It Will Last Forever."

Studies now show that about one-third of people with IBS will lose their symptoms and complaints over time for reasons that are not understood. This offers hope for many people with IBS, because spontaneous improvement can occur with time. Still, this is not the case for everybody. Proper diagnosis and understanding of the MindBodySpirit Connection can help most people with IBS live a more normal life.

## "You're Just Stressed, Anxious or Depressed."

You now understand that a disturbance in the MindBodySpirit and Mind/Brain-Gut Connection is responsible for the symptoms of IBS and other functional symptoms and syndromes. You know that you must think systemically rather than linearly to understand IBS. While the problem is not "just stress," it is not appropriate to trivialize the role stress plays in illness and disease. The consequences of the bad stress response and allostatic load are harmful, not only relative to generation of functional symptoms and syndromes, but also in the contribution to and causation of serious diseases, such as Metabolic Syndrome X.

You can think of anxiety and depression as symptoms that have a similar origin to that of functional symptoms and syndromes. This is why anxiety and depression are so commonly associated with the diagnosis of IBS. It is important that anxiety and depression be properly diagnosed, since treatment can contribute to overall symptom relief and clear the way for healing.

## "IBS Is Colitis."

Unfortunately, many patients (and even some doctors) use the term *colitis* when they really mean IBS. This causes confusion, because colitis is a disorder in which the inner lining of the colon is inflamed. Common causes of colitis are infections and inflammatory bowel diseases like ulcerative colitis and Crohn's disease (see Chapter 14). There is no colitis or inflammation in IBS. The terms *colitis* and *spastic colitis* are misnomers.

## "IBS Can Lead to Cancer."

There is no relationship between IBS and colon cancer. IBS does not increase the risk of developing colon polyps and cancer. But because the symptoms of IBS can sometimes cover up symptoms of colon cancer, it is a good idea to have regular screening examinations for colon polyps and cancer. See Chapter 14 for more information about colorectal polyps and cancer.

## "I Will Need a Lot of Tests to Find Out What's Wrong."

In Chapter 14, you learned how doctors diagnose IBS. They use positive symptom diagnosis in order to reduce the number of tests that are necessary.

In the next chapter, you will learn about dietary triggers and dietary issues in IBS.

# Chapter 16
## *Diet and IBS*

Unfortunately . . . a dietary approach to the irritable bowel
syndrome has not, in the majority of cases, solved the patient's
discomfort. . . . Now the emphasis has shifted to the increased
sensitivity of the patient's nerves, transferring the origin of
symptoms from the gut to the brain.
– *Good Food for Bad Stomachs*
Henry D. Janowitz, M.D.
Gastroenterologist Emeritus
Mount Sinai School of Medicine

Eating healthy, balanced, regular meals slowly and in a pleasant environment is essential to taking good care of yourself. Avoidance of
a few common dietary triggers may be beneficial, but most of the
time, placing undue emphasis upon dietary restrictions is not particularly helpful in relieving the symptoms of IBS. Keeping a diary
of the foods you eat and how you react to them may be more useful. If your symptoms persist, additional dietary suggestions are included for you in this chapter and in Chapter 17, where we discuss
dietary fiber.

## Common Internal Triggers/Stressors

Table 11.1 in Chapter 11 listed some of the common internal triggers/
stressors of IBS, some of which involve various foods. For this reason,
dietary changes may be helpful in relieving IBS symptoms, particularly if
symptoms appear to be associated with ingestion of common triggering
substances.

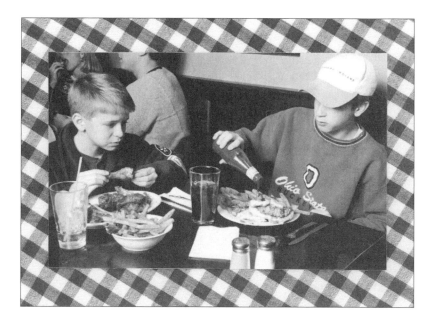

- **Fat.**    Fat—especially saturated fat—can trigger cramping and the sudden need to have a bowel movement and diarrhea by stimulating the release of chemical messenger molecules that promote gut contractions. Furthermore, bloating and distention can be triggered by fat. Finally, fat can also aggravate nausea, heartburn (GERD) and dyspepsia by slowing stomach emptying and aggravating gastro-esophageal reflux.

- **Lactose.**    The milk sugar lactose is a carbohydrate that is found in milk and dairy products. Lactose malabsorption is very common—particularly in Asian Americans, Native Americans, African Americans and Hispanic Americans. Lactose intolerance is caused by too little lactase, the enzyme that breaks down lactose in the digestive tract lining. Lactose intolerance is usually dose-related, meaning that most people with lactase enzyme deficiency can tolerate some dairy products (unlike a true milk allergy), especially if taken with a meal. Scientific study has shown a poor correlation between reported lactose intolerance and true lactose malabsorption and the common failure of lactose restriction to improve symptoms. A two-week trial restricting milk, frozen yogurt, ice cream and soft cheese (especially mozzarella and cottage cheese) is usually sufficient to determine whether lactose intolerance is contributing to symptoms.

- **Sorbitol.**   Sorbitol is a sugar found naturally in certain fruits. It is also used as an artificial sweetener. Sorbitol is very poorly absorbed, even in people who do not have IBS. The larger the dose, the greater the problem with absorption. Foods and products that contain sorbitol include:
  - Some elixir (liquid) medications, in which the sorbitol may be called an "inactive ingredient"
  - "Sugarless" candy, breath mints and chewing gum
  - Apples, pears, prunes and peaches
  - Fruits canned in concentrated apple or pear juice, often labeled "Light" or "Lite"
  - Fruit juice drinks
- **Caffeine.**   Caffeine is a stimulant of the Mind/Brain-Gut Connection that can contribute to abdominal cramping and diarrhea. Furthermore, caffeine can aggravate anxiety, which in turn can contribute to digestive tract symptoms in a vicious cycle.
- **Alcohol.**   Some people are very sensitive to the triggering effects of alcohol. Symptoms include cramping, diarrhea, dyspepsia and heartburn. Alcohol can also disrupt sleep, which further contributes to imbalance and disturbance of the Mind/Brain-Gut Connection.
- **Indigestible carbohydrates.**   Certain foods contain a complex carbohydrate called raffinose, which is incompletely absorbed and can trigger IBS symptoms and flatulence. Foods that are high in raffinose include beans, cabbage, Brussels sprouts, broccoli and asparagus.
- **Fructose and hydrolyzed corn syrup.**   Fructose is the natural sugar in sweet fruits, honey, onions and artichokes. Fructose is also manufactured by treating corn with enzymes, which yields a synthetic honey called "corn sweetener" or "corn syrup." Fructose is used as a sweetener in some soft drinks and fruit drinks.
- **Wheat.**   Wheat is a grain found in most breads, crackers, pasta and many other foods. Two different problems associated with wheat can occur. First, some people seem to have a wheat intolerance that

triggers symptoms of cramping, abdominal distention, bloating, flatulence or diarrhea. This is not a true allergy, but restriction of wheat and wheat-containing products may help to relieve symptoms.

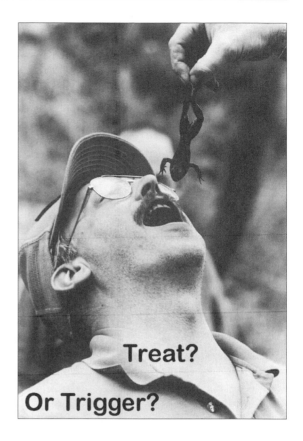

Treat? Or Trigger?

Second, some people have celiac sprue (also known as gluten-sensitive enteropathy or non-tropical sprue), which is a disorder caused by a specific sensitivity to gluten. Gluten is the protein component of wheat, barley, rye and oats that imparts the sticky character to dough. It can cause a true allergic reaction that damages the wall of the intestine. This results in impaired fat and nutrient absorption. Celiac sprue is an important condition to rule out before diagnosing IBS, particularly if symptoms include diarrhea or weight loss, or if iron deficiency anemia is detected on blood testing (see Chapter 14).

- **Fiber.**    Fiber can be a triggering substance for some patients with IBS. However, many people, patients and doctors underestimate the potential health and symptom benefits of fiber, especially if symptoms of constipation are present. Chapter 17 includes a detailed discussion about fiber and how to include it in the diet.

- **"Natural" remedies (see later discussion).**    Anthraquinone derivative laxatives (Chapter 18) may be included in many "natural" remedies that are advertised as colon health products, herbal laxatives and even teas. These "natural" products may or may not identify the laxative as an ingredient. If it is identified, the laxative may be described as harmless and "natural," such as locust plant or *Cassia angustofolia* (senna). Thus, some people taking a "natural" remedy may be taking a stimulant laxative unknowingly, which can trigger IBS symptoms.

# Chronic Diarrhea

A scientific study reported that the most common triggering foods and substances for functional diarrhea include wheat products, dairy products, citrus fruits, eggs, onions, nuts, caffeine and alcohol (*Gut*, 1989;30: 1099–1104). Sorbitol is another potential trigger for diarrhea (see earlier discussion).

# Abdominal Bloating and Distention

The symptom of abdominal bloating and distention was discussed in Chapter 13. Scientific studies confirm that eating fats can markedly increase abdominal discomfort perception and lower the discomfort threshold for distention. So, bloating and distention may increase and be more painful after large, fatty meals. Fiber may aggravate the symptom of bloating without an associated excess of flatulence. Restriction of "gas forming" foods may or may not be helpful.

# Flatulence

Gas and flatulence are discussed in Chapter 13. Most foods that contain carbohydrates can cause flatulence. These have been discussed earlier in this chapter and include lactose, sorbitol, indigestible carbohydrates (raffinose), fructose, wheat and fiber. Most starches also result in gas production as they are digested. These include potatoes, corn, noodles and wheat. *Rice is the only starch that is not associated with gas production.*

Many people are concerned about malodorous, or bad-smelling gas. Foods and substances that are potentially odor forming may include alcohol, asparagus, beans, cabbage, chicken, coffee, cucumbers, dairy products, eggs, fish, garlic, nuts, onions, prunes, radishes and highly seasoned foods.

# Food Intolerance

Fifty percent of people believe that they have some food intolerance(s). While patients with IBS very commonly suspect food intolerances, dyspepsia or other functional gut disorders, scientific proof of offending foods has been difficult to obtain. Elimination diets to identify specific food intolerances are difficult and interpretation of results can be controversial. It is often impossible to distinguish true physical food intolerance from a conditioned response and psychological aversion. As you learned earlier, it may simply be the mechanical presence of food as an internal gut stressor that triggers symptoms, rather than specific foods per se.

# Elimination Diet

An elimination diet requires that you eliminate most foods from your diet initially while maintaining a careful diary. Food groups are then gradually reintroduced into the diet, and you observe and record your reactions in the diary. An elimination diet may help you identify unsuspected triggers.

*If you try an elimination diet, remember the following:*
- Keep a careful diary.
- Do not rely upon your memory. If you are going to go to the trouble of trying an elimination regimen, then you must take the time to record your reactions in writing and analyze them afterward.
- Psychological stressors and emotional upset might be playing an important role in your symptoms. Therefore, you might incorrectly implicate a food when the problem is really that symptoms are occurring in relationship to your stress response. This is why a diary in which you also include your emotional state of mind can be helpful.
- Prepackaged and processed foods can contain unsuspected triggering foods and substances. There are some exceptions, such as carefully prepared organic foods, but a good rule of thumb to remember is, "fresh is best."
- The amount of food eaten may matter. In other words, small amounts of a food may not be a problem, while larger amounts may. So make note of the quantity of food that you eat.

- Some foods may only act as a trigger when eaten alone and not when eaten with other foods.
- Strictly avoid alcohol, caffeine and coffee during the elimination diet trial.

There is no single elimination diet that has received a consensus of acceptance. If you wish to consider an elimination diet, here are our suggestions.

## Core diet

Henry Janowitz, M.D., is a well-known gastroenterologist from New York who recommends the "core diet" in his book, *Good Food for Bad Stomachs*. He has over 20 years of experience with this simple—although very restricted—elimination diet and maintains that it is very rare to be sensitive to these initial foods (Table 16.1).

---

Table 16.1

### Janowitz "Core" Diet

1. Bottled mineral water without carbonation
2. One starch (rice). Instant rice or raw rice can be cooked with mineral water
3. One protein (either boiled, broiled or roast chicken or broiled lamb chops, but not both)*
4. One fruit (he recommends canned Bartlett pears)

---

*If you are a vegetarian, substitute soy for a protein source (soymilk or tofu), even though occasionally individuals have difficulties digesting soy.

The diet should be followed for at least two weeks while symptoms subside. Then a new food can be added every day, with egg, wheat and milk as the last to be added. If a reaction is produced by a new addition, it is then necessary to "back up" to the previous level where your symptoms were controlled or resolved and start again after a week of stabilization.

## Another exclusion diet

A British scientific study with only a small number of women suggested that some with IBS might have disturbances in bacterial gas fermentation and colonic gas production (*Lancet,* 1998;352:1187–1189). An exclusion diet was used: fish and meat (except beef) were allowed, but dairy products were replaced with soy products, and cereals other than rice were forbidden. There were also restrictions placed on yeast, citrus fruits, caffeinated drinks and tap water. Symptoms (stool frequency and looseness with abdominal pain and flatulence occurring daily) were reduced on the exclusion diet.

## Suggestions about food reintroduction

*Milk.*   Milk should be reintroduced as skim milk, so there is no question about whether fat in milk is the problem. If skim milk can be consumed without symptoms, then the problem is clearly not related to milk in any way.

*Wheat.*   Wheat can be eaten as a whole-wheat cereal and whole-wheat bread. Other grains, like barley, oats and corn, can be added.

*Cooked versus raw.*   Cooked fruits and vegetables may be better tolerated initially than in uncooked form. Later, you can try them raw if they do not cause symptoms when cooked.

# Food Allergy

There is a considerable industry based upon pseudoscience and misinformation about food allergies. More than 25% of Americans believe that they or their children are allergic to specific foods. But true allergic reactions to food occur in no more than 2% of adults and 8% of children. Many more people actually have food intolerances, as discussed previously. There is a definite need for more research on food allergies.

## Chronic hives (urticaria)

Some people have chronic and recurrent hives, or urticaria. However, studies show that less than 1% of cases are caused by a food allergy.

## If you suspect food allergy

If you suspect that you have a food allergy, follow these three steps.

*First, ask yourself three questions.*

1. *What are my symptoms?* Symptoms of allergic reactions are distinctive: itching, hives, eczema, irritated and itchy eyes, tightness in the throat, wheezing, cough, nausea and vomiting and diarrhea.

2. *Do the symptoms occur within 30 minutes of eating?* The longer the time between eating and onset of symptoms, the less likely that the symptoms are coming from a food allergy. True allergic reactions occur within 30 minutes and often immediately after eating. The key is to keep a food diary for several weeks, as discussed earlier in this chapter.

3. *Have the following foods that are most likely to cause true allergic reactions in adults been considered?* The most common foods that can cause an allergic reaction include hen's eggs, peanuts, tree nuts, fish, shellfish or crustaceans (shrimps, scallops and crab), soy, gluten (the protein of wheat, barley, rye and oats), food additives (particularly colorings and dyes) and cow's milk protein. The allergen in milk and milk products is the protein casein. A wide range of foods may contain some form of casein or other milk proteins, including hot dogs, bologna, canned tuna, sorbet and tofu or rice-based desserts. True cow's milk allergy occurs in about 4% in children. Allergy to milk proteins is very rare in adults compared to lactose malabsorption and intolerance.

*Second, check the Food Allergy & Anaphylaxis Network.*   The Food Allergy & Anaphylaxis Network has an Internet site that offers patients and health-care professionals news and education about food allergies: www.foodallergy.org.

*Third, consider a hypoallergenic diet.*   If a true food allergy is suspected, a hypoallergenic diet can be tried for 2 to 3 weeks (Table 16.2). This approach is usually not helpful with food intolerances, since true allergy to dietary substances is rare in adults. If a benefit is evident, then new foods can be gradually introduced to attempt identification of the offending food type or dietary substance. An allowed food should be avoided if it has caused a reaction in the past. Maintain a record during the elimination diet, and if symptoms occur, check to see if there is any relationship to particular foods.

Table 16.2

**Sample Elimination (Exclusion or Hypoallergenic) Diet**

| Food Category | Allowed | Avoid |
|---|---|---|
| Meat and meat alternatives | Lamb, chicken and turkey | Pork, beef, fish, eggs, milk and milk products, seafood |
| Grains | Rice, tapioca, arrow-root | Wheat, oats, corn, rye |
| Legumes and nuts | None | Avoid all dried peas, beans and nuts |
| Vegetables | All except → | corn and peas |
| Fruits | All except → | citrus fruits, strawberries and tomatoes |
| Sweeteners | Sugar (cane or beet), maple syrup, honey | Avoid all artificial sweeteners |
| Fats and oils | Olive oil, safflower oil, Crisco | Soy, corn, peanut oils, butter, margarine |
| Miscellaneous | White vinegar, water, salt, fruit juices | Coffee, tea, alcohol, chocolate, colas, spices, chewing gum |

## Treatment of food allergy

Other than avoidance, there are no effective treatments for food allergies. If allergies are confirmed, you should carry an epinephrine kit at all times; exposure to hidden allergens in foods thought to be safe is fairly common. Even if the epinephrine eliminates the initial symptoms, immediate medical attention should be sought.

# Olestra (Olean®)

In response to the emphasis upon reducing the amount of fat in the diet, the no-calorie fat replacer called olestra (OLEAN®, Procter & Gamble, Cincinnati, OH) was developed to help people reduce the amount of fat they eat. OLEAN® is made from table sugar and vegetable oil. The OLEAN® molecule is too large to be digested or absorbed, so it adds no fat or calories. For example, a 1-ounce bag of potato chips made with OLEAN® contains 0 grams of fat and about 70 calories, while full-fat potato chips have 10 grams of fat and 150 calories. OLEAN® looks, tastes, cooks and seems like fat. Scientific studies do not suggest that digestive tract side effects with OLEAN® are any more likely than they would be with full-fat foods.

Learn what you need to know about dietary fiber in the next chapter.

# Chapter 17
## *Fiber*

Most people should strive for a daily fiber
intake of from 20 to 35 grams per day.
*– Nutrition and Your Health: Dietary
Guidelines for Americans*

Adequate dietary fiber can be helpful in treating IBS, particularly if
the symptom of constipation is present. Most people in the United
States only eat 10 to 15 grams of fiber each day, even though current
dietary recommendations call for eating 20 to 35 grams of fiber per
day. Most people and patients—and many doctors—do not empha-
size adequate dietary fiber intake enough and do not understand
how to incorporate fiber into the diet.

## Definition of Fiber

Fiber includes all of the complex plant carbohydrates that are not digested
or absorbed in the small intestine. This includes whole-grain breads and
cereals, beans, peas and other fruits and vegetables. Once fiber enters the
colon, bacteria in the gut digest it in a process called fermentation. Several different types of fiber with different chemical structures and differ-
ing abilities to dissolve in water have been identified, but it is most useful
to think of fiber as either soluble or insoluble. Both types of fiber are important for healthy digestive function.

### Soluble fiber

Soluble fiber disperses well in water and liquid and forms a soft gel in the
digestive tract. It is not broken down until it reaches the colon, where its

digestion and fermentation causes the production of gas. Examples of soluble fiber are oats, barley, beans, peas and many types of fruit.

### Insoluble fiber

Insoluble fiber does not disperse in water and liquid and undergoes only minimal change as it passes through the digestive tract. Examples of insoluble fiber include wheat bran, whole-grain breads and many vegetables.

# Fiber and the Gut

Fiber is necessary to promote normal peristalsis, the wavelike muscular contractions that move food along the intestinal tract. As fiber passes along, it absorbs water, which softens and bulks up the stool. Higher stool bulk results in softer and larger stools for most people and eases the elimination of stool. With more bulk, pressure in the colon is actually reduced—it does not have to contract as strongly to propel the stool along. This is important for people who have constipation, since most will benefit by increasing dietary fiber intake. This point cannot be stressed enough. In fact, some constipated people may require more fiber than the recommended 20 to 35 grams per day. Severe forms of constipation may not respond to fiber and require other forms of treatment.

Some people with chronic diarrhea benefit by increased fiber intake, as fiber absorbs water from the stool and increases consistency. The fiber supplement psyllium may be particularly beneficial (see later discussion on fiber supplements).

Increased fiber intake can relieve symptoms of hemorrhoids and difficulty cleansing the anal area by improving stool consistency and frequency and by reducing the adherence of stool following defecation. Again, psyllium seems to be especially helpful here.

Finally, diverticulosis of the colon is correlated with low dietary fiber intake (see Chapter 14). A high fiber intake can actually reduce the pressure within the colon and is particularly helpful if constipation is also present. Contrary to popular belief, there is no evidence that small seeds and grains, nuts and popcorn cause complications from diverticulosis.

# How Much Fiber Should I Take?

The United States has one of the lowest dietary fiber intakes per capita in the world. The average American only takes in 13 grams of fiber per day. By contrast, Africans take in an average of 60 grams of fiber per day. Health experts now recommend that most people should increase dietary fiber intake to 20 to 35 grams per day. For most people, this means at least doubling the daily fiber intake. Some people with constipation benefit by eating even more fiber than the recommended amounts. As you read the goals of fiber intake, remember that the normal bowel pattern in the United States is from three bowel movements per day to three bowel movements per week.

*The goal of fiber intake should be:*
- At least three soft bowel movements per week
- Comfortable passage of soft stool without undue straining
- Avoidance of harsh stimulant laxatives

One of Bill's retired partners, Eugene May, M.D., used to tell his patients to eat enough fiber so that their bowel movements were "totally tubular and the diameter of a quarter." We think that this is good advice!

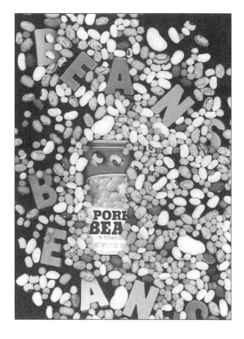

# How to Increase Dietary Fiber

You can easily increase dietary fiber by eating more whole grains. Look for cereals that provide at least 4 to 5 grams of fiber per serving. Whole grain breads are far superior to products made from white flour.

You can also increase your consumption of fruits (especially berries) and vegetables (especially beans). For example, add dates, figs or prunes to the serving of cereal in the morning. Dried fruits such as cherries, blueberries and apricots can be taken to work and eaten as a snack. Cooked beans of all types are a good source of fiber. They provide approximately 4 to 5 grams of fiber per half-cup serving. Learn more about <u>increasing dietary fiber</u>.

## Add fiber gradually and be consistent

It is usually best to gradually increase fiber intake over the course of several weeks to reduce the chance of developing cramping, bloating and flatulence. Most people find that the symptoms caused by eating more dietary fiber gradually decline over one to two months. Furthermore, the relief from constipation or diarrhea is an acceptable trade-off. It is important to be consistent by ingesting adequate dietary fiber each day. Symptoms may be aggravated if dietary fiber intake is irregular.

## Drink adequate amounts of water and fluids

It is important to drink plenty of water and fluids when dietary fiber is increased. Try to drink six to eight 8-ounce glasses of fluid each day.

## Take fiber supplements

It can be difficult to meet the recommended fiber intake of 20 to 35 grams per day through your diet. If this is the case, consider utilizing dietary fiber supplements. Several products are available.

*Psyllium,* derived from grinding the seeds of a species of plantain *(Plantago psyllium),* is an excellent source of soluble as well as insoluble fiber. Psyllium is the main ingredient of many commercially available bulk products, such as Hydrocil, Konsyl, Fiberall, Metamucil and Perdiem. Psyllium is generically available and powdered psyllium seed can be purchased at groceries and health food stores. A good starting dose is between 3 to 6 grams stirred or shaken in a glass of water or juice, followed by another glass of fluid. *Psyllium is the only fiber supplement that has received approval by the Food and Drug Administration for lowering cholesterol when taken in conjunction with a low-fat diet.*

*Methylcellulose* (brand name is Citrucel) is a semi-synthetic soluble fiber that does not undergo bacterial fermentation and breakdown. This may result in fewer problems with flatulence, even though scientific studies have not confirmed a benefit over psyllium in this regard.

*Calcium polycarbophil* (brand names are Equalactin, FiberCon and Mitrolan) is a synthetic fiber that is not fermented and broken down by bacteria. It acts as an insoluble fiber.

### Flaxseed

Flaxseed is an inexpensive source of fiber and omega-3 fatty acids, which is a healthy type of fat discussed in Chapter 26. Flaxseed can be found in health food stores and some supermarkets. If they are eaten whole, the seeds pass through the digestive tract undigested. Flaxseed must be ground (as in a dedicated coffee grinder) in order to release the omega-3 fatty acids. They can be ground and sprinkled upon foods. An average serving size of these pleasant, nutty-tasting seeds is ¼ cup (48 grams), which contains 140 calories and 6 grams of fiber. Flaxseed is best stored in the refrigerator. If it is purchased ready-ground, it is susceptible to decay.

# If Symptoms Worsen or Develop

Remember to introduce fiber gradually, as was discussed earlier. Try to remain optimistic that your symptoms will diminish or disappear over the following month. However, be aware that some patients with IBS have a significant problem with abdominal bloating and flatulence when they increase the fiber content of the diet and do not seem to be able to adjust to the change. Because of an increased sensitivity to what is happening in the digestive tract, gas released by the breakdown and fermentation of the complex carbohydrates of fiber causes distention of the colon that is perceived as discomfort, bloating and pain. Furthermore, some people are more likely to produce gas than are others. If bran causes gas and flatulence, try concentrating on eating more whole grains, fruits and vegetables. Review Chapter 16 on diet. Fiber supplements can be tried, and some products may be better tolerated than others.

In the next chapter, you will review medical treatment with both prescription drugs and "natural" complementary/alternative therapies for functional gut symptoms and IBS.

# Chapter 18

## *Treatment of IBS and Other Functional Gut Syndromes*

It's really a very simple idea: no prescription
is worth more than knowledge.
– C. Everett Koop, M.D.
Former Surgeon General of the United States


In such a night
Medea gathered the enchanted herbs
That did renew old Aeson.
– Shakespeare

---

Your IBS has placed you on a path to healing through an understanding of your MindBodySpirit/Brain-Gut Connection and Mind-
BodySpirit medicine. You now understand how important improving the health of your mind, body and spirit is to improving your
IBS symptoms. However, if you need or prefer to take treatment
with drugs, medications or "natural" therapies, then this chapter can
be your treatment guide.

---

## First . . .

You are beginning to appreciate that you can change the way you understand and respond to your symptoms and become healthy. You know that
treatment and healing are not the same. Perhaps you had been searching
for a treatment cure of your IBS. Unfortunately, such a treatment or pill
is not likely in the near future. However, some effective medications are

available now, and new scientific understanding of the neurobiology of the Mind/Brain-Gut Connection has led to active research in pursuit of drug treatments that can help relieve IBS symptoms. New treatments will come.

If you and your doctor decide that treatment is advisable now, be sure to learn as much about the medications and/or "natural" remedies as you can. This chapter is a guide to treatment options for IBS and other functional syndromes. It is not intended to replace the information you receive from your doctor, your pharmacist, drug inserts and other reliable sources. Also understand that all potential side effects of treatments are not included here.

# The Science of Medical Treatment for IBS

Jailwala, Imperiale and Kroenke have written a review of scientific studies published up to the year 2000 on drug treatment of IBS (*Annals of Internal Medicine,* 2000;133:136–147). These researchers concluded the following:

- Antispasmodics/smooth muscle relaxant drugs are beneficial when pain is the predominant symptom.
- Loperamide (brand name Imodium; generic drugs available) is effective for diarrhea but not for pain.
- Bulking agents (Chapter 17) improve constipation and stool consistency but do not improve pain.
- Chinese herbal medications and other medications that have been studied sporadically and in small trials need to be further investigated before specific conclusions can be drawn.
- Some antidepressant drugs appear to be effective in the treatment of some of the symptoms of functional gut disorders.

Additional studies support the value of antispasmodic drugs for the treatment of abdominal pain (*Alimentary Pharmacology & Therapeutics,* 1994; 8:499–510 and 2001;15:355–361).

## Treatment Focuses on the Symptoms

Medical treatment for patients with IBS is usually directed to the predominant symptoms, which include abdominal discomfort and pain, diarrhea, constipation and bloating/distention (Drossman D.A., Whitehead W.E., Camilleri M., et al. "Irritable Bowel Syndrome: A Technical Review for Guidelines Development." *Gastroenterology,* 1997;112: 2120–37).

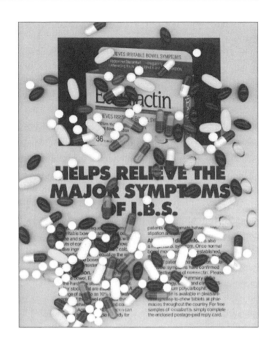

### Abdominal discomfort and pain

When the main symptom of IBS is abdominal pain, drug choices include antispasmodics, analgesic drugs (non-narcotic and narcotic), antidepressant drugs (see later discussion) and newer 5-HT drugs (see later discussion).

*Antispasmodics.*   There are three classes of antispasmodics, or drugs that decrease gut contraction and spasm.

1. **Anticholinergics** work by blocking the effects of the parasympathetic branch of the autonomic nervous system (one of the Mind-BodySpirit communication systems described in Chapter 7). Examples include dicyclomine (Bentyl is a brand name), hyoscyamine (brand names Anaspaz, Levsin, Levsinex and NuLev), glycopyrrolate (brand name Robinul), methscopolamine bromide (brand name Pamine) and propantheline (a brand name is Probanthine). One drug (a brand name is Librax) is an anticholinergic drug called clidinium combined with a benzodiazepine antianxiety drug called chlordiazepoxide. Another (brand names Donnatal and

Donnatal Extentabs) combines two anticholinergic drugs called atropine and scopolamine with a barbiturate antianxiety drug called phenobarbital.

2. **Direct smooth muscle relaxants** act directly upon the smooth muscle of the gut. Studies show that the direct smooth muscle relaxants may be the most effective of the antispasmodics, but these drugs are not available in the United States. Examples of direct smooth muscle relaxant drugs include octylonium, mebeverine and trimebutine.

3. **Peppermint oil** is thought to work by decreasing calcium entry into muscle cells, resulting in muscle relaxation. Enteric-coated preparations may be preferable to unprotected peppermint because they allow delivery of the peppermint oil to the colon. Peppermint oil may or may not be effective. Scientific studies of the oil's use are inconclusive.

*Analgesic drugs.*    Analgesic drugs are either non-narcotic or narcotic.

• *Non-narcotic.*    Non-narcotic analgesic drugs (aspirin, acetaminophen, nonsteroidal anti-inflammatory drugs, also known as NSAIDS) are usually of little benefit in treating the abdominal pain of IBS. Tramadol (brand name Ultram), is a non-narcotic analgesic drug that binds to opiate receptors in the brain and alters serotonin and norepinephrine reuptake, which inhibits the transmission of pain signals to the brain through ascending pathways from the body and gut. It is best to begin with a very low dosage and gradually increase it over several days to reduce the likelihood of unacceptable side effects (mainly nausea).

• *Narcotic.*    Narcotic analgesic drugs are usually not prescribed for continuous treatment because of possible development of physical dependency or addiction and unwanted side effects, such as drowsiness and interference with clear thinking. Furthermore, continuous narcotic use can actually increase pain sensitivity and also alter gut motility, leading to severe constipation. This is called the "narcotic bowel syndrome" (*Annals of Internal Medicine,* 1984;101:331–334). Keeping these cautions in mind, narcotic analgesic drugs are occasionally used to relieve intermittent attacks of more severe pain.

## Diarrhea

There are two main functional gastrointestinal disorders where diarrhea is a prominent symptom: (1) chronic functional diarrhea and (2) the more common diarrhea-predominant IBS, or D-IBS (see Chapters 13 and 14).

Treatment choices include the opioid agonists loperamide (a brand name Imodium; generic available) and diphenoxylate (a brand name Lomotil; generic available). Diphenoxylate also contains atropine, which is an antispasmodic discussed earlier.

Two drugs that are used to lower blood cholesterol can be helpful for some patients with chronic diarrhea, especially if the problem tends to occur in the morning, is triggered by meals or develops after surgical removal of the gallbladder. These drugs are cholestyramine (brand name Questran; generic available) and colestipol (brand name Colestid; generic available).

Narcotic drugs, such as codeine, are opioid agonists and have constipation as a potential side effect, so they may relieve diarrhea. However, because they cross into the brain, they can have unwanted side effects of sedation and drowsiness, and they can lead to physical dependency and addiction (see earlier discussion of narcotic analgesics).

Unless a dietary factor can be identified as a trigger or cause of chronic diarrhea (Chapter 16), opioid agonists are usually recommended first. Studies show that loperamide reduces the urgency and frequency of bowel movements in patients with diarrhea-predominant IBS. Furthermore, loperamide can increase stool consistency and strengthen anal sphincter tone, which can be helpful if fecal incontinence is a problem. Loperamide does not get into the brain through the blood-brain barrier and is usually preferred over other opioids, such as codeine or diphenoxylate. However, none of these agents have been shown to relieve the pain associated with IBS. The drugs can either be taken regularly or on a prophylactic basis. If a "morning rush" occurs (Chapter 13), then the drug could be taken at bedtime.

A study has shown that tricyclic antidepressant drugs (TCAs) may relieve diarrhea and associated pain in some patients with IBS, in part by their anticholinergic effects. Refer to the preceding discussion on "Anticholinergics" and to the later discussion on "Antidepressant Drugs."

## Constipation

There are two functional gut disorders where constipation is a prominent symptom: (1) constipation-predominant IBS, or C-IBS and (2) functional constipation (see Chapters 13 and 14). **Remember that the normal frequency of bowel movements ranges from three per day to three per week.**

When constipation is the predominant symptom, the first step for most patients is a trial of adequate dietary fiber intake. Additional options include laxatives and medications.

*Dietary fiber and fiber supplements (bulk agents or bulk laxatives).* Most people, including doctors, do not appreciate the potential benefits of adequate fiber intake and how to incorporate fiber into the diet. Review Chapter 17 for details. Most who have mild to moderate uncomplicated constipation improve when fiber intake is increased. Those who either fail to respond to increased fiber intake, cannot tolerate it or require additional help may need to utilize laxatives.

*Laxatives.*    There are two types of laxatives, osmotic and stimulant. Osmotic laxatives are not absorbed and most require a prescription. They soften the stool and have an onset of action of one to three days. One type of osmotic laxative is polyethylene glycol, or PEG (a brand name is Miralax). Another is unabsorbed carbohydrate (lactulose and sorbitol). Glycerine suppositories are available without prescription.

Stimulant laxatives interfere with absorption and motility and are available without prescription. They have an onset of action of six to twelve hours and produce a soft to semi-fluid stool. They include saline laxatives (brand names Milk of Magnesia and Citrate of Magnesia); diphenyl-methane derivatives (brand name Dulcolax); and anthraquinone derivatives (senna, cascara sagrada and aloin).

Anthraquinones are widely available. They may also be included in many "natural" remedies (see later discussion) that are advertised as colon health products, herbal laxatives and even teas. These laxatives may or may not be identified in the list of ingredients. If they are identified, they may be described as harmless and "natural," such as locust plant or *Cassia angustofolia* (senna). Make sure to tell your doctor if you are taking one of these products.

• *Chronic use of laxatives.*   The belief that stimulant laxatives can damage the colon is probably untrue. This is the conclusion drawn by Dr. Arnold Wald, a gastroenterologist at the University of Pittsburgh Medical Center, who is an expert on constipation. We agree with his recommendations that chronic use of laxatives is not harmful when they are used appropriately. Remember that most people with constipation can be adequately relieved with adequate dietary fiber intake. Osmotic laxatives can be used on a daily basis. If necessary for symptom relief, stimulant laxatives should be used no more often than two to three times weekly (*4th International Symposium on Functional Gastrointestinal Disorders,* March 30–April 2, 2001, Milwaukee, WI).

### Bloating and distention

No drug therapies have been confirmed to benefit bloating and distention; however, antidepressant drugs may help (see next section on Antidepressant Drugs). A recent study suggested that patients who took one capsule of pancreatic enzyme supplement prior to eating high-fat meals (brand name Creon 10; available by prescription) significantly minimized their abdominal bloating, flatulence and nausea (*Digestive Diseases and Sciences,* July, 1999).

# Antidepressant Drugs

Antidepressants are commonly prescribed for IBS and other functional gut and bodily symptoms and syndromes, even though the Food and Drug Administration (FDA) does not specifically approve them for this purpose unless depression is present. This is called an "off-label" indication. Nevertheless, antidepressants can be helpful in bringing symptom relief in IBS and other functional syndromes, such as fibromyalgia (*American Journal of Medicine,* 2000 Jan;108(1):65–72; *Journal of General Internal Medicine,* 2000 Sep;15(9):659–66). If depression is present, then a full antidepressant drug dose is necessary. If depression is not present, then lower doses may be effective.

At Digestive Disease Week 2001 in Atlanta, Georgia, University of North Carolina gastroenterologist Douglas A. Drossman said that, "The use of antidepressants in IBS and other GI disorders is growing." When symptoms become repetitive, severe and/or are associated with alteration in quality of life, antidepressant drugs can be considered.

Antidepressants have effects on gut motility (contractions) and sensation and also may have pain modulatory benefits. Antidepressant drugs are not addictive. Table 18.1 gives examples of antidepressants in each of three classes. Brand names are given in parentheses.

Table 18.1

### Classes of Antidepressant Drugs

| Tricyclics (TCAs) | Selective Serotonin Re-uptake Inhibitors (SSRIs) | Unique Property Antidepressants |
|---|---|---|
| Amitriptyline (Elavil) | Citalopram (Celexa) | Buproprion (Wellbutrin) |
| Clomipramine (Anafranil) | Fluoxetine (Prozac) | Mirtazepine (Remeron) |
| Desipramine (Norpramin) | Fluvoxamine (Luvox) | Nefazedone (Serzone) |
| Doxepin (Sinequan) | Paroxetine (Paxil) | Trazodone (Desyrel) |
| Imipramine (Tofranil) | Sertraline (Zoloft) | Venlafaxine (Effexor) |
| Nortriptyline (Pamelor) | | |

## Questions for you and your doctor

Antidepressant drugs may be of benefit in the treatment of abdominal pain and discomfort associated with IBS; however, the tricyclic antidepressants (TCAs) have proven to be more effective than the selective serotonin reuptake inhibitors (SSRIs) in the small number of scientific studies that have been conducted. The efficacy of SSRIs in treatment of functional gut syndromes such as IBS is currently being investigated. In clinical practice, finding the best drug is often a matter addressing several important questions:

- *Are you depressed, along with your digestive symptoms?* If so, then an antidepressant drug dose will be needed, because the presence of depression can magnify and amplify your symptoms. If you are not depressed, then lower antidepressant drug doses may be effective.
- *Do you have previous experience with antidepressant drugs?* If a drug helped before, it may be wise to select the same one again. But, if a specific antidepressant was not helpful before or caused unacceptable side effects, then it doesn't make much sense to try it again.
- *Do you have concerns about taking antidepressants?* If you have taken antidepressant drugs previously, inform your doctor about which drug or drugs that you have taken, whether they helped or whether they caused unacceptable side effects. Also, discuss any reluctance that you may have regarding taking antidepressants. The purpose of treatment with an antidepressant drug is to help you to feel better and not to alter your mind adversely. Antidepressant drugs are not addictive.
- *Do you also have other functional symptoms and/or syndromes, such as fibromyalgia and interstitial cystitis?* If so, then antidepressant drugs may be helpful in reducing or relieving more than just the digestive symptoms.
- *Do you have a family member or family members who have benefited from a specific antidepressant or had unwanted side effects?* Remember what you have learned about your family history. You may want to take this into consideration when you and your doctor select an antidepressant.
- *Do you have any significant health problems, especially with your heart and circulation, liver and kidneys?* For example, it may be important to avoid the TCAs if you have heart arrhythmia.
- *What are your predominant symptoms?*
  - **Pain or discomfort:** TCAs may be the best initial choice.
  - **Diarrhea:** some antidepressants have constipation as a side effect and could be helpful for diarrhea.
  - **Constipation:** some antidepressants are more likely to cause diarrhea, which might improve the constipation. TCAs have not been

shown to be beneficial in treatment of constipation and may either cause or aggravate the condition.
- **Sleeping problems:** some antidepressants are more helpful in promoting sleep than others, and some may actually interfere with sleep.
- **Sleepy or sluggish:** some antidepressants can boost energy.
- **Nervous or jittery:** some drugs can bring a calming effect.

## Be patient

It can take several weeks for an antidepressant to take effect. If treatment is stopped too soon, then it may appear that the treatment did not work. If you experience side effects, discuss them with your doctor. Most side effects will either diminish or go away completely after several days, or they can be reduced temporarily by lowering the dose. Furthermore, the decision to continue treatment or consider a change of medication can be re-evaluated at a later appointment. Since everyone is different, trying one or more different antidepressant drugs may be necessary in order to find the one that is best for you.

## Unwanted side effects

Space will not permit a detailed discussion of potential antidepressant drug side effects, but a common one is sexual dysfunction. Unfortunately, some of the antidepressant drugs interfere with sexuality and sexual function by reducing libido or causing difficulty with achievement of erection or orgasm. The antidepressant drugs that are less likely to cause this problem are buproprion (brand name Wellbutrin), mirtazepine (brand name Remeron), Nefazedone (brand name Serzone) and possibly citalopram (brand name Celexa).

# Antianxiety Drugs (Anxiolytics)

Anxiety may be associated with IBS. If so, then antianxiety drugs, called anxiolytics, may be helpful.

## Benzodiazepines

Benzodiazepines are commonly used in the treatment of anxiety, but they can cause drowsiness, sedation, memory impairment and interactions with other drugs and alcohol. Furthermore, physical dependency can develop, so that physical withdrawal symptoms and rebound anxiety can occur upon discontinuation. It is for this reason that discontinuation of long-term benzodiazepine treatment requires a slow tapering of dose. Finally, benzodiazepines may cause or aggravate depression. For these reasons, they are usually prescribed only when anxiety is moderate to severe. The most commonly prescribed benzodiazepines (brand names in parentheses) are clonazepam (Klonopin); diazepam (Valium); lorazepam (Ativan); and alprazolam (Xanax). Generic versions of each are available.

## Buspirone (brand name is BuSpar)

Buspirone is a non-benzodiazepine drug that is approved for treatment of chronic anxiety. It is less likely to cause drowsiness and sedation than benzodiazepines, but dizziness and nausea can occur during initial treatment.

## Antidepressant drugs

Antidepressant drugs can be used in the treatment of anxiety (see "Antidepressant Drugs").

# Newer Drugs

Newer drugs have been developed that are agonists (drugs that enhance) and antagonists (drugs that block) the effects of the neurotransmitter 5-HT (serotonin) in the gut (see Chapter 7). Learn more about new drugs for IBS.

## Diarrhea-predominant IBS

Alosetron (brand name Lotronex) is a 5-HT3 antagonist used to treat diarrhea-predominant IBS in women (it has not been shown to be effective in men during research). It was withdrawn from the U.S. market in 2000 because of concerns over its safety. The most common side effect was constipation, but a type of colon inflammation called ischemic colitis was found to be associated with, although not definitely caused by, the drug.

## Constipation-predominant IBS

Tegaserod (brand name Zelnorm) is a 5-HT4 agonist designed to treat constipation-predominant IBS. It should be a promising treatment for C-IBS, but it has not yet been approved for use in the United States by the FDA. Scientific studies have shown that if side effects do occur, they are minor (headache, diarrhea). No cases of ischemic colitis have been reported.

# "Natural" Remedies

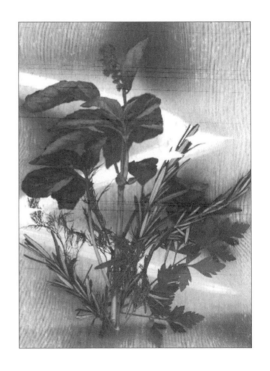

The placebo response is evidence of the remarkable self-healing capacity that we all have. Howard Brody, M.D., is a physician at Michigan State University who has written a book called *The Placebo Response: How You Can Release the Body's Inner Pharmacy for Better Health.* He defines the placebo response as "a change in the body (or the body-mind unit) that occurs as the result of the symbolic significance that one attributes to an event or object in the healing environment." You will learn about this in detail in Step 4. As UCLA gastroenterologist Dr. Emeran Mayer has written, "If we are honest with ourselves, treatment practices do not necessarily have to be better than placebo to find a useful place in medical practice, and honest practitioners have used this approach to the benefit of their patients for many years. Conversely, practitioners who eschew the healing arts in favor of only offering their patients scientific evidence-based therapies may be justifiably accused of doing their patients a serious disservice" (*The Neuro-*

*biology Basis of Mind Body Medicine,* The International Foundation for Functional Gastrointestinal Disorders, 2001).

Most of the evidence for efficacy of "natural" remedies and herbal products is empirically derived, which means that recommendations and usage are based upon repeated experience and observation throughout history. Few have been subjected to the rigors of scientific testing. But even if no better than placebo, "natural" remedies may bc helpful. Numerous products are now available, marketed as daily dietary supplements, in accordance with the Dietary Supplement Health and Education Act (DSHEA). DSHEA products carry nutrition support statements that may include

---

### General Recommendations about "Natural" Medicines and Herbals

If you decide to take natural remedies or herbal medicines, here are our recommendations.

- Don't take them if you don't need them.
- You may need to experiment with herbal remedies, since most of the evidence for efficacy is empirical, meaning that recommendations and usage are based upon repeated experience and observation throughout history. Few have been subjected to the rigors of scientific testing. Allow your experience to be your guide and use only those remedies that provide you with consistent benefits.
- Be sure to let your doctor know about it, particularly since some of these treatments can react with prescription drugs.
- Herbal products may be contaminated or adulterated, and they may not contain advertised amounts of the active ingredients. So, purchase reputable brands that also advertise the purity of their ingredients. Search for herbal preparations that have been "wildcrafted" (harvested from wild stands) or cultivated organically.
- Discontinue use if you have an adverse reaction.
- Tinctures (alcohol based) and freeze-dried extracts of herbals are usually the best preparations to purchase.
- Loose herbs that are sold in bulk and powdered herbals within capsules are less likely to be effective.

---

claims regarding the effects of the product on the structure or function of the body. In doing so, they must carry the following disclaimer: *"This statement has not been evaluated by the Food and Drug Administration. This product is not intended to diagnose, treat, cure or prevent any disease."*

This chapter provides an introduction to some specific recommendations regarding "natural" therapies, considered to be complementary/alternative medicines.

## Products

Here is a brief description of some of the most commonly used "natural" remedies and herbal products.

*Acidophilus.*    Acidophilus is a probiotic (see later discussion) that consists of dried or liquid cultures of live bacteria that sour milk and are considered beneficial or "friendly" to the GI tract. Health food stores carry acidophilus in preparations that have much higher concentrations of the bacteria than are found in yogurt and acidophilus milk.
*Used for:* IBS, diarrhea or to avoid diarrhea when taking antibiotics

*Aloe or aloe vera.*    The clear gel from the aloe plant is used in many skin lotions, creams and cosmetics because of its moisturizing properties. Aloe vera juice, sold in health food stores, can be taken internally. If the dose is too high, it can have a laxative effect. A reasonable amount to try is 1 teaspoon after meals. The fresh gel can be mashed up in fruit juice. There is variation in palatability, so it may be necessary to try different brands.
*Used for:* Inflammatory bowel disease (Crohn's disease and ulcerative colitis)

*Aromatherapy.*    The five senses send information to the limbic system. Aromatherapy is based upon the fact that sense of smell is the only sense that is wired directly into the limbic system. Scents that are purported to be helpful in IBS include peppermint, eucalyptus, lavender and rose oil. A certified aromatherapist ensures use of essential oils and not synthetic chemicals.
*Used for:* IBS

*Beano (brand name).*    Beano is manufactured by AKPharma, Inc., the manufacturers of Lactaid and Prelief. Beano contains an enzyme called alpha-galactosidase that digests the indigestible carbohydrate (raffinose) contained in beans and some vegetables. Beano has no effect on gas associated with other carbohydrates, such as sorbitol, lactose, wheat and fiber. It cannot be added to food while it is being cooked, since heat degrades the enzyme.

*Used for:*  Flatulence

***Calcium glycerophosphate (brand name Prelief).***    The manufacturer of Prelief, AKPharma, Inc., advertises that, "Prelief takes acid out of food. Prelief reduces the acid in all food and beverages so you can enjoy a more comfortable diet."

*Used for:*  Food sensitivity, IBS, interstitial cystitis

***Chamomile.***    Chamomile is the dried flowers of the perennial chamomile plant. It is available as an extract, oil and tea.

*Used for:*  Nausea, dyspepsia, IBS, anxiety

***Charcoal.***    Activated charcoal tablets or capsules (brand names include Charco Caps and Charcoal Plus) may help provide relief from flatulence by reducing intestinal gas.

*Used for:*  Flatulence

***Chinese herbal medicine.***    Chinese herbal medicine has been used in China for centuries in the treatment of IBS symptoms. A recent scientific study published in the *Journal of the American Medical Association* (1998;280:1585–1590) concluded that Chinese herbal medicine may be beneficial in the treatment of IBS. The product used was supplied by Mei Yu Imports.

*Used for:*  IBS

***Chlorophyllin copper.***    Products that contain chlorophyllin copper (brand names include Nullo and Derifil) may help to reduce the offending odor of flatus.

*Used for:*  Malodorous flatulence

***Fennel.***    Fennel *(Foeniculum vulgare)* includes the seeds, leaves and roots of the fennel plant. It is available in plain seeds, sugar coated seeds, extract, oil and capsules. The adult dose is one half-teaspoon of fennel

seeds chewed after eating or whenever symptoms are bothersome, or as recommended on the product label.
*Used for:*  Rectal gas and flatulence

*Flaxseed.*   Refer to Chapter 17 for more information.
*Used for:*  Source of fiber and omega-3 fatty acids

*Ginger.*   Ginger is a spice that is available in fresh form from supermarkets, as candied ginger, honey-based ginger syrups, tinctures and powdered extract in capsules.
*Used for:*  Nausea, dyspepsia

*Kava.*   Kava is a derivative of a plant indigenous to the South Sea Islands *(Piper methysticum)* that has a mild relaxant and antianxiety effect.
*Used for:*  Anxiety

*Lactase enzyme.*   Brand names of products containing lactase enzyme for lactose intolerance include Lactaid, Dairy-Ease and Lactrase. Refer to Chapter 16 for more information about lactose intolerance.
*Used for:*  Lactose intolerance

*Passion flower.*   Passion flower is an herbal made from a Native American plant *(Passiflora incarnata)* that has a mild relaxant effect.
*Used for:*  Anxiety

*Peppermint.*   Peppermint is available in capsules that have a protective coating that resists digestion by the stomach acid so that the peppermint can be released in the colon. There are several brands available, but we recommend the brand names of Mintacin or Peppermint Plus (manufactured by Enzymatic Therapy, Inc; www.enzy.com).
*Used for:*  IBS

*Probiotics.*   "Probiotic" is the term used to describe health-promoting "friendly" bacteria ingested orally. These bacteria in the intestine purportedly provide a protective effect only when a proper balance is maintained among all the different bacteria that normally reside in the intestine. If normal bacteria become depleted or the balance is disturbed by diet, infection, antibiotic use, lifestyle changes or stress, then potentially harmful "unfriendly" bacteria can overgrow and become established, leading to digestive and other health problems. These harmful bacteria are alleged to have the ability to cause gastrointestinal problems such as diarrhea, abdominal pain and/or bloating if not kept in check by the beneficial bacteria. Furthermore, probiotics supposedly promote digestive health, balance and function and help maintain a healthy balance of "good" bacteria in the digestive tract.

Probiotics are credited with an impressive list of therapeutic and prophylactic attributes. The probiotics industry is flourishing, and interest in establishing scientific credibility has attained importance for many companies and scientists. Probiotics are the subject of considerable scientific research. For now, if you decide to try a probiotic, the most commonly recognized probiotics are the lactic acid bacteria that include lactobacilli, streptococci and/or bifidobacterium. Some commercially available products include *Lactobacillus acidophilus* (many brands available); *Lactobacillus reuteri* (brand name Probiotica), manufactured by McNeil, the company that makes Imodium; *Lactobacillus GG* (brand name Culturelle), made by CAG Functional Foods—a ConAgra Company; and *Saccharomyces boulardii*.
*Used for:* A variety of gut symptoms and digestive health

*SAMe (s-Adenosyl methionine).*   This dietary supplement is a prescription drug for depression in Europe, but it is available in the United States without prescription and promoted as a natural product for the treatment of depression or arthritis. SAMe contains an important compound that is produced by all living cells, which is involved in the regulation of several hormones and neurotransmitter chemical messengers, such as serotonin and epinephrine. SAMe is expensive.
*Used for:* Depression (not severe or associated with suicidal ideation) and arthritis

*Simethicone.*   Simethicone is a foaming agent that joins gas bubbles in the stomach, which may increase the amount of gas that can be belched away. Brand names include Gas-X, Mylanta Gas and Phazyme. Simethicone has no effect on intestinal gas.
*Used for:* Belching

*Slippery elm.*    Slippery elm is obtained from the inner bark of the red elm tree and is said to restore the normal mucus coating on irritated tissues. Slippery elm lozenges can be found in most grocery stores.
*Used for:* Inflammatory bowel disease (Crohn's disease and ulcerative colitis)

*St. John's wort.*    St. John's wort *(Hypericum perforatum)* may be useful in treating depression, although scientific studies are inconclusive.
*Used for:* Depression (not severe or associated with suicidal ideation)

*Triphala.*    Triphala is an Ayurvedic Indian mixture used to treat constipation and poor bowel tone. Indian practitioners of Ayurvedic medicine recommend two Indian brands: Dabur and Hammdar. The dose is two capsules per day or as recommended by the manufacturer.
*Used for:* Constipation and poor bowel tone

There is a distinction between treatment and healing. This chapter addresses treatment. But keep in mind that you have a new and positive language— MindBodySpirit Medicine—to help you heal.

*Valerian.*    Obtained from the root of an European plant, *Valeriana officinalis* was the main sedative and hypnotic in use in Europe and America before the invention of barbiturates in the early twentieth century.
*Used for:* Sleep aid

# References and Resources

Learn more about <u>complementary and alternative medical treatments for IBS</u>.

Take the next step and choose to heal.

# STEP 4

## CHOOSING TO HEAL

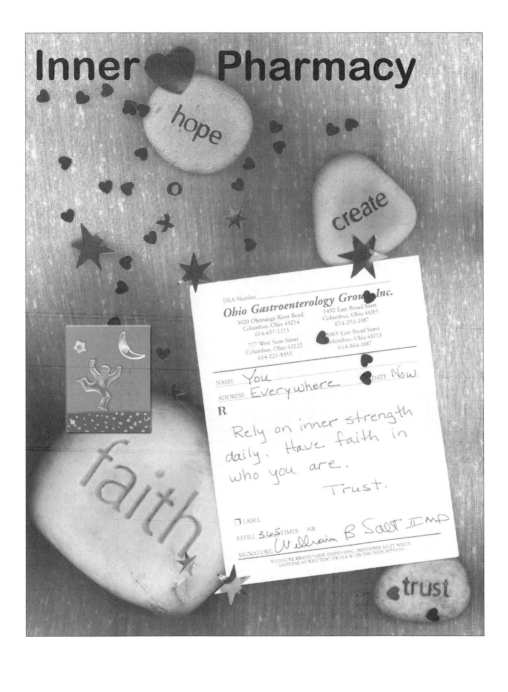

# Chapter 19
## *The Healing Response*

Of one thing I am certain, the body is not the
measure of healing, peace is the measure.
— George Melton

The unexamined life is not worth living.
— Socrates

Healing is anything that moves us towards a greater sense of physical, emotional, mental and spiritual well-being. In its essence, healing is a yearning, an impulse towards our own wholeness and an intentional movement towards peace of mind, body and spirit. Though a cure is not always possible for people with IBS, some measure of healing is possible for almost everyone.

## Finding a Cure

When you are faced with a serious medical problem or chronic disturbing symptoms like those of IBS, you hope that a reliable cure exists for your condition. A cure looks like this: you go to your doctor, who listens to your symptoms, diagnoses your problem, pulls out a prescription pad and scribbles the name of a medicine that only your pharmacist can decipher and fill. Then, after taking your pills for the prescribed period of time, your problem is gone; you are cured.

In simple conditions like a strep throat, middle ear infection or nausea from a stomach flu, this scenario works. Unfortunately, IBS and other functional symptoms, syndromes and most chronic recurring medical problems do not respond so cooperatively to a single medicine or even to multiple attempts at treatment. In this regard, there is no cure. This can be frustrating, but don't give up hope. Even when a cure is not available, healing is.

# Beyond a Cure and into the Healing Response

What is meant by the word *healing?* The Latin root for *healing* means, "to be whole." In essence, healing is a yearning and an impulse towards our own wholeness and fullness of being. Although seeking out a cure is a vital step in healing, it is only a part of the larger whole. Healing is a process and an intentional movement toward peace of mind, body and spirit.

Even when a cure is not possible, healing is, because you can almost always find ways to improve your mental, emotional and spiritual health, in spite of physical illness. Healing as an intentional process implies that you are capable of responding to your pain through a series of clear and intelligent steps that give you some level of control and mastery over how well your body heals. To better understand the healing process, let's look for a moment at the process by which a cut to the skin heals.

## Physical healing

When you cut your skin, pain draws your awareness to the cut. In that awareness, you clean the wound and apply an antibacterial salve to fight off infection. Then you place a bandage on the cut to help bring the edges of the wound together and keep it protected. Days later, you remove the bandage and the cut is almost completely healed.

This simple process of wound healing is amazing. All you need to do is be willing to bring the edges of the wound together and keep it clean and protected. By your intelligent participation, you aid the healing process by helping to create the proper environment for healing, but "you" are not doing the healing. In its inner wisdom, your body knows how to heal. Bernie Siegel, M.D., author and surgeon, says, "I cut into the body and I rely on it to heal. I don't have to yell into the wound and tell it how to heal."

This is one of the fundamental principles of all MindBodySpirit healing: the healing system lies within us. This means that the body has its own natural ability to heal. In certain situations, surgery or drugs may be life saving, but it is the internal healing system that most often keeps us alive.

## Intentional healing

Let's review the steps that promote physical healing. We can use them as a model to understand the steps toward total healing not only of the body, but also the mind and spirit. The first step toward healing a cut in the skin is the awareness of pain. Pain is something most people instinctively shy away from, but without pain no healing would be possible. Once you are aware of pain, you can bring your focused attention and knowledge to the task of healing the cut. You take directed and educated steps to clean and protect the wound and bring the edges together, thereby transcending the isolation—the separation—created by the cut. All these steps are necessary for what Elliot Dacher, M.D., calls "intentional healing" in his book, *Intentional Healing.* He calls for directing the power of your mind toward the healing process. Intentional healing may be directed toward emotional and spiritual healing as well as physical healing.

## Emotional healing

Emotional healing is anything that helps you to transcend the isolation you feel in your life because of unresolved anger, sadness, hurt, loss, fear or disappointment. To heal emotionally, you must bring the edges of the emotional wound together by taking intelligent steps towards processing the feelings that are creating your sense of isolation.

How do you bring the edges of an emotional wound together? How do you process the feelings that cause you emotional pain? By reaching out to a friend, therapist or counselor; by spending time in the presence of someone who loves you; by making peace with the one who hurt you; or by finding a place of understanding, forgiveness or acceptance. In these ways, you begin the process of "removing" the painful feelings that keep your emotional wound open, thereby reconnecting the edges of the wound and allowing the healing to begin.

## Spiritual healing

Spiritual healing is about finding a connection to something greater than yourself, be it friendship, community, a sense of virtue or meaning, God, a higher power or some sense of higher truth, beauty or sacredness in life. Spiritual healing, therefore, is anything that helps you to transcend the isolation you feel because of a lack of meaning or purpose in life, or because of a lack of connection to a higher power or sense of something greater than yourself.

There are two main methods of spiritual healing. First, find and nurture some connection with a *higher purpose* in life, a sense that your life has meaning and value to yourself and others. Second, find and nurture some connection to a *higher power* in your life. Your higher purpose and higher power are united by an affirmative answer to the question, "Is what I am thinking, doing or saying going to lead me to greater love, kindness and compassion?" All spiritual healing leads to the fruit of greater love and acceptance—of yourself and others.

Let's look at some of the limitations of the old model of medicine in light of these new concepts of healing. This will help you understand how the new model—MindBodySpirit medicine—can help you find relief from your IBS.

# Limits of Modern Medicine

Elliott Dacher, M.D., in his book *Intentional Healing,* discusses the limits of modern medicine. He proposes a new model that explores the frontiers of healing made possible through MindBodySpirit medicine. The old model of medicine involves the doctor asking for your symptoms, making a diagnosis and then choosing a treatment (usually a medication, surgical procedure, dietary recommendation or physical therapy) to cure or alleviate your symptoms. In this old model, your "ticket of admission" into the medical system is a symptom that causes you pain and suffering.

The problem with this biomedical model is that it focuses almost exclusively on the *symptoms* of disease and overlooks the deeper—and most often hidden—causes of your symptoms. The deeper causes of your symptoms often arise from the invisible world of thought, feeling, attitude and belief, which lead to unhealthy lifestyles. These lifestyle choices contribute greatly to disease symptoms.

## Treatment: Reaching Out, Reaching In

All forms of healing (physical, mental, emotional and spiritual) require you to focus simultaneously on two complementary aspects of treatment: (1) *reaching out* for the best that medical science has to offer and (2) *reaching in* to mobilize your own internal resources for healing.

*Reaching out* involves the use of any external agent or intervention (like drugs, surgery, radiation, diet, physical therapy, herbs, counseling or support groups) to help alleviate the symptoms—or lead to the cure—of the underlying disease. Most old-model, disease-oriented approaches to illness focus on these external treatments. However, in today's rushed world of managed care, these "reaching out" treatments are usually directed at the reduction or elimination of symptoms alone, with limited attention given to underlying lifestyle choices, and little or no attention given to psychological and spiritual factors associated with illness.

*Reaching in* involves the use of any internal resource or intervention (like meditation, journaling, will-power, positive belief, healthy expectations or prayer) to help alleviate the symptoms—or lead to the cure—of the underlying disease. "Reaching in" treatments imply the use of your natural capabilities—of the inner power and resources of your mind, body and spirit—to restore health. Herbert Benson, M.D., refers to this aspect of treatment as "self-care," and believes that it can improve the effectiveness of almost all external (reaching out) forms of treatment.

In order to better understand how you can utilize this information to help you heal your IBS, let's look at Dr. Dacher's new model for healing, called the "Whole Healing System."

## The Whole Healing System

In his book, *Whole Healing,* Elliot Dacher describes a practical method for applying the MindBodySpirit model of health and healing. It gives you a logical and systematic approach to developing a healing program for your IBS symptoms. The Whole Healing System model is composed of four independent but interrelated healing systems that comprise the whole person. The independent healing systems are spiritual, mind/body, treatment and homeostatic (Figure 19.1). 🖥 Learn more about the Whole Healing System.

## The Whole Healing System

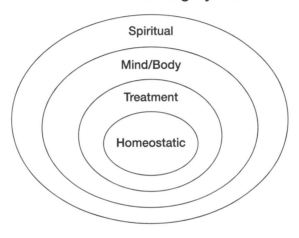

**Figure 19.1**
Reprinted with the permission of Elliott S. Dacher, M.D., from his website, www.healthy.net.

1. *The Homeostatic Healing System* is the *built-in, instinctual* system of internal physiologic and biochemical checks and balances that maintain health through the dynamic process of allostasis described in Step 2. When threatened by perceived triggers/stressors, the homeostatic healing system is designed to restore stability through change. The "good stress" response is adaptive. The "bad stress" response is maladaptive.

2. *The Treatment Healing System* involves the application of "reaching out" treatments, like drugs, surgery, radiation and "natural" remedies, to help restore health when the homeostatic healing system fails. The treatment healing system is symptom—and disease—oriented, focused on curing illness and restoring function

159

      rather than promoting health. This system is most often *culturally determined* (i.e., "Western medicine" versus "Eastern/Oriental medicine") and varies in different cultures.

3. *The Mind/Body Healing System* draws on the use of *intentionally activated* knowledge and awareness to address personal attitudes, stressful lifestyles and psychological beliefs that may be contributing to ill health. This system assumes a level of personal responsibility and self-motivation for achieving health. Dr. Dacher says that, "the concern here is with psychological development, individuation, personal transformation, and mastery, to the extent possible, over the activities of the mind and body." The major treatments involve "reaching in" through meditation, yoga and biofeedback and "reaching out" through exercise, nutritional practices, support groups, stress management and health education.

4. *The Spiritual Healing System* involves changes in consciousness and connectedness that create a sense of peace, wholeness and belonging. Whereas the mind/body healing system is intentionally activated, spiritual healing is *intuitively discovered* through insight, prayer, meditation and self-reflection. This system focuses on the meaning of health and illness and the narratives you create to explain the events of your life.

## Applying These Concepts to Your IBS

Let's look at how Dr. Dacher's Whole Healing System can help you with your IBS. In this system, you and your doctor would pursue relief for you through all four of the healing systems.

When you first visit your physician with symptoms of abdominal pain, cramping and constipation or diarrhea, your doctor listens to your symptoms and after an examination and possibly some laboratory or imaging studies, arrives at a diagnosis of IBS. The fact that your laboratory tests are basically normal insures the relative integrity of your *homeostatic healing system.* So you and your doctor will move on to the *treatment healing system,* in which you will be given a trial-and-error series of drugs, dietary recommendations and herbal remedies in an attempt to relieve your symptoms. Remember, you are a partner in this process. If treatment at this level succeeds, you will probably proceed no further. However, if your symptoms continue to disrupt and control your life, then you would proceed to the *mind/body healing system* for help, while continuing to work with your doctor.

You would examine particular lifestyle choices, stressors/triggers, attitudes, thoughts and beliefs that could be contributing to your physical symptoms and distress. Although you would be working with your doctor, perhaps with the help of a therapist, psychologist or psychiatrist, you would actively participate in your own treatment and assume responsibility for mind/body healing. Then if you could not find the comfort and relief that you desire, you would move on to the next level of healing, the *spiritual healing system.*

At this level, you will require the continued support of your doctor as a healing resource, but you may also require the help of a spiritual counselor (pastor, priest, rabbi, guru or mentor) to help you navigate the realms of consciousness, meaning and connectedness. At this level you will begin to intuitively discover your own narratives about illness and health, pain and suffering, life and meaning. As you probe the depths of consciousness and discover who you are and what gives your life meaning, purpose and transcendence, you will begin to experience greater spiritual peace and health.

In the next chapter we will look at how your attitudes, beliefs and expectations influence your physical health.

# Chapter 20

## *Your Choices Define You*

We are all co-creators of reality . . . our goal in life is not just to be bright, alert or imaginative, but to shape existence itself. It becomes every person's choice to take responsibility for his own inner reality.
– Deepak Chopra, M.D.

**The human mind converts our ideas and expectations into biochemical realities.**
– Norman Cousins

You have the ability—and the responsibility—to choose your attitudes and beliefs. What you choose to believe is no less vital to your health and healing than what you choose to eat and drink. The power of belief lies in the realm of the invisible world of thought and feeling, but the mind, through processes still being discovered, converts these attitudes, beliefs and expectations into biochemical realities. Thus, your choices define who—and what—you are.

Attitudes and beliefs have everything to do with how you experience life, both in difficult and in joyous times. Attitudes and beliefs, like seeds buried in the deep earth, give rise to trees that bear fruit. Your positive beliefs bear the fruit of greater love, compassion and health. Your negative beliefs bear the fruit of fear, isolation and illness. Positive attitudes empower you to focus on the blessings in your daily life and to enjoy a measure of happiness that you might otherwise overlook if you focus only on the difficulties in your life.

*Having a positive attitude does not mean pretending to be happy or upbeat.* Rather, it is about having a mature outlook that recognizes your true blessings even in the midst of the sadness, pain and loss inherent in a full and vital life. Developing positive attitudes and beliefs is an acquired skill. It can be learned by even the most cynical and hostile among us! Cultivating positive attitudes and beliefs—as well as eliminating negative attitudes and beliefs—is a vital part of healing your IBS.

## Three Premises About Attitudes and Beliefs

When it comes to understanding how your attitudes and beliefs affect your physical health and your symptoms of IBS, it is important to understand three basic premises:

1. You have the ability—and the responsibility—to choose your attitudes and beliefs.
2. Positive attitudes and beliefs are empowering and increase your capacity for health, happiness and peace of mind. Negative attitudes and beliefs are disempowering and diminish your capacity for health, happiness and peace of mind.
3. The attitudes and beliefs you hold represent forces of the human mind that are no less powerful than a physician's prescription pad.

We will examine each of these three premises in detail through the rest of Step 4.

## Premise 1: You Have the Ability to Choose Your Attitudes and Beliefs

The fundamental starting point for harnessing the healing power of your attitudes and beliefs is the realization that you have the ability to choose them. Viktor Frankl, M.D., a psychiatrist and Holocaust survivor who wrote *Man's Search for Meaning*, says, ". . . everything can be taken from a man but one thing; the last of human freedoms—to choose one's attitude in any given set of circumstances, to choose one's own way."

The difficulty is that many of the beliefs and attitudes you hold were chosen *for* you, not chosen *by* you. They were chosen for you by your parents, your teachers and your incorrect assumptions about life experiences. Many were chosen for you when you were too young to draw your own conclusions about life.

## "Define or be defined"

In the animal world, there is a saying: "Eat or be eaten." In the spiritual world, the saying is: "Define or be defined." In other words, if you fail to define who you are and what you believe, others will be glad to do it for you! An illness such as IBS may define you. Hopelessness may define you. You have the ability to choose the attitudes and beliefs that define you and the responsibility to choose them wisely. What you choose to believe affects your attitudes, your behaviors and the very fabric of your physiology and biochemistry.

## "Both/and" and "either/or" thinking

Picture this cartoon. We'll refer back to it in later discussions:

> One caveman has just ignited a spark by rubbing two sticks together. He has discovered fire! The other caveman is a reporter. He pulls out his hammer and chisel to record the event on a stone slab. He turns to the man who has just discovered fire and asks, "How shall I refer to you, as the discoverer of fire or as the first person to pollute the atmosphere?"

Which one is it? Which belief do you choose? The choice is yours. But before you choose, consider the concept of "both/and" thinking. "Both/and" thinking allows the caveman above to be *both* the discoverer of fire *and* the first polluter. The ability to perceive *both* good *and* bad, black and white, and right and wrong allows you to develop a spiritual maturity with which to confront life's difficulties. Maturity may be defined as the ability to see the many shades of gray that exist in the world. The concept of "both/and" allows you to see the complexities of life while still choosing to follow those beliefs and values that are most empowering to you.

The opposite of "both/and" is "either/or." "Either/or" thinking forces you to make false choices. Life is *either* good *or* bad; the caveman is *either* the discoverer of fire *or* the first polluter. Both cannot be true and there is no middle ground to stand on. "Either/or" choices deplete your energy and often lead to polarization, stubbornness of opinion and quick judgments about people and situations. "Either/or" thinking ignores the complexities of life and impairs your ability to achieve greater empathy, understanding, love and forgiveness.

## Choosing Beliefs and Attitudes

Many beliefs you hold are based upon your perceptions of life—what you perceive to be true. Perceptions are nothing more than the things you become aware of through your senses. The conclusions you then draw about your perceptions are called "beliefs." The problem with basing your beliefs upon your perceptions is that perceptions are often incomplete and your senses can be easily tricked.

The set of conclusions and beliefs you draw about your life or your illness make up what is called "the story" or "the narrative" of your life or illness. You will learn in the upcoming chapters about the ways in which the meaning you attach to "the story" of your life or illness effects your very physiology and biochemistry. For now, understand that nearly all life events present you with many options about what to believe. What you choose to believe dramatically affects your ability to overcome illness, endure the pain necessary for growth and healing, and achieve the sense of happiness and peace of mind that is so vital to a life well lived.

## You See What You Look For

Let's do a little experiment. Take 30 seconds and look around the room where you are now sitting and look for everything that is blue. *Stop reading now and do it!*

Okay, are you done? Did you find everything blue in the room? Great! Now, take 30 seconds and write down everything in the room that is red! Yes, red! Here's the point: What you choose to see in any given circumstance is heavily influenced by what you are looking for. If you are looking for everything blue in the room, you are going to notice the blue. If you are looking for the blessings in your life, that is what you are going to notice. If you are focused on the pain, discomfort and lack of control you seem to have over your IBS, that is what you are going to notice. If you are focused on the progress, peace and joy in your life, you will be less likely to suffer from the pain and discomfort of your IBS.

Please understand that this does not mean you are to pretend that you do not have pain, cramping, diarrhea, constipation and other disturbing symptoms. They are real and no amount of pretending will take them away. But, you can realize that at the same time that there is pain, cramping, diarrhea and constipation in your life, there is also joy, happiness, friendship and peace in your life. The good and the bad coexist. Without denying one or the other, you can choose which world you will focus on. Over that, you have complete control.

## Perceptions and Beliefs

Your collective beliefs make up "the story" of your life or illness, and are often based on your perceptions. In order to change the story of your illness for the better, you need to understand the sometimes-circular relationship that exists between your perceptions and beliefs.

Imagine that you are in charge of videotaping a party. Your eyes and ears are like the lens and microphone of the camera. What gets recorded on videotape is similar to what you see and hear (your perceptions) at the party. You can expand your perceptions (what you see and hear) by pointing your camera in a different direction or by changing the lens of the camera in order to zoom in or zoom out of a situation. Your beliefs represent what you as the videographer choose to film—where you choose to point your camera.

Figure 20.1 shows how your beliefs color what you see by leading you to look only for those things that support what you expect to find or believe to be true. In this respect, you only see (perceive) what you believe to be true. Because your beliefs color your perceptions and your perceptions confirm your beliefs, you tend to get stuck.

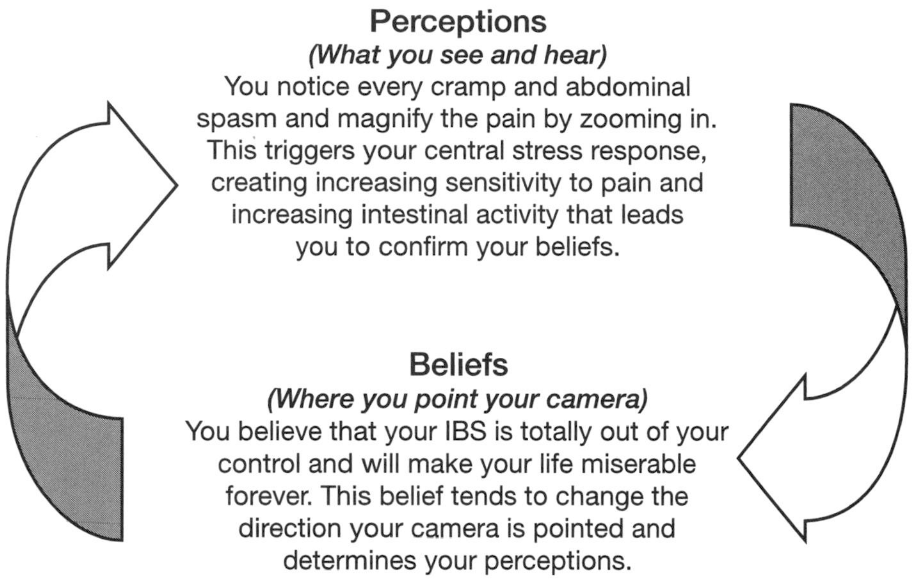

## Perceptions
### *(What you see and hear)*
You notice every cramp and abdominal spasm and magnify the pain by zooming in. This triggers your central stress response, creating increasing sensitivity to pain and increasing intestinal activity that leads you to confirm your beliefs.

## Beliefs
### *(Where you point your camera)*
You believe that your IBS is totally out of your control and will make your life miserable forever. This belief tends to change the direction your camera is pointed and determines your perceptions.

**Figure 20.1**
Reprinted with the permission of Neil F. Neimark, M.D.

You can break this cycle with "both/and" thinking—you can work on both changing your beliefs and expanding your perceptions. When you do this, you begin to realize that changing your beliefs can expand your perceptions and that expanding your perceptions can change your beliefs. Let's examine in more detail how you can do this.

## How beliefs limit perceptions

If you believe that you don't "fit in" with certain people at the party, you will tend to associate with those people you do fit in with. When you do this, you limit or narrow your perceptions (what you see or hear) to one small segment of the party. In other words, the videotape of your life is "stuck" on a small segment of the party. Because you *believe* you don't "fit in" with certain people or situations, you miss out on all the other conversations going on at the party. If you can change your belief that you don't fit in, then you can expand your perceptions by visiting with (videotaping) more people at the party. In this way, changing your beliefs expands your perceptions.

### How perceptions limit beliefs

The reverse is also true: expanding your perceptions can change your beliefs. Let's say that you are with a small group of people at the party and the conversation is stale and boring. After a short while, you think to yourself, "this party is boring. I'm going to leave." But just then, you hear some laughter from another corner of the room and look over to see a bunch of old friends you didn't know were there. You politely excuse yourself, greet your old friends and end up having a great time at the party. In this case, your expanded perceptions (i.e., seeing your old friends and hearing their laughter) changed your beliefs about the party. It was no longer boring.

You control the camera of your life, the movie of your life, the story of your life. You can direct the camera toward any of an infinite number of scenes. At any given moment, there are many things to be grateful for and many things to be upset about. Where are you going to point your camera?

Learn more about <u>perceptions</u>.

## Counting Blessings

One of the best ways to expand your perceptions and empower your beliefs is to look for the blessing in everything that happens to you. What if "everything"—even things that that don't seem to turn out for the best—carries with it some benefit? What if it is your job to discover, learn and grow from it? Wouldn't that change the way you view your IBS, stress and adversity? If you look for a blessing in every experience, if you look for a way to heal and grow, some of your suffering may be alleviated.

Looking for the blessing in everything that happens is really about looking for the possibilities for growth, freedom and healing in every situation. Though certain life events may seem at first to hinder your growth, limit your freedom or sabotage your health, you can often find within those events the seeds of even greater growth, freedom and healing. In what ways does IBS hinder your growth, limit your freedom and sabotage your health? Now ask yourself if your IBS has—in some way—made you more loving, stronger or more compassionate with others. Can you find within your IBS the seeds of greater growth, freedom and healing?

When you think of—and focus on—the possibilities in life, the words of Norman Cousins come to mind, when he said, ". . . no one really knows enough to be a pessimist. There are too many imponderables out there to be able to say that something can't be done. And so I've learned to respect the imponderables and that means respecting the possibilities."

This kind of "possibility thinking" is powerful and healing. Remember that no one really does know enough to be a pessimist. There is always a possibility for hope and a possibility for love, even when certain things are taken from you. What are the possibilities for love, growth and healing that may be contained within your struggle with IBS? What are the blessings contained in your struggle with IBS? Learn more about <u>counting blessings</u>.

Let's move on to the next chapter where we'll discuss how positive attitudes increase your capacity for health, happiness and healing.

# Chapter 21

## *Positive Attitudes Heal*

"Positive attitudes are no guarantee of a cure, but they can improve
the quality of life and generate the most out of what is possible."
– Norman Cousins

Positive attitudes and beliefs are empowering and increase your capacity for health, happiness and peace of mind. Negative attitudes and beliefs are disempowering and diminish your capacity for health, happiness and peace of mind. In this chapter, we'll look at how positive attitudes increase your capacity for health.

## Premise 2: Positive Attitudes and Beliefs Increase Your Capacity for Health

Carl Simonton, author of *Getting Well Again,* found in a study of 152 cancer patients that "a positive attitude toward treatment was a better predictor of response to treatment than was the severity of the disease." This means that recovery from illness involves much more than the biology and biochemistry of the disease. Attitudes and beliefs exert a powerful moderating force on the disease process itself. The biology of the disease and the biology of the individual interact with each other in disease development, maintenance and recovery. The attitudes and beliefs you hold contribute to the make up of your unique individual biology.

Let's look at how two different attitudes and beliefs might affect your response to treatment.

*Belief #1:* IBS arises from genetic and environmental factors outside your control and there is very little you can do to get better.

*Belief #2:* IBS arises from a combination of genetic predisposition and the bad stress response, and with proper knowledge, you can dramatically lessen the severity of your symptoms and improve the quality of your life.

What you choose to believe is critical. You can see that your choice will dramatically influence your attitude about your illness; the strength of your conviction to practice behaviors that can help you overcome IBS; and most importantly, your sense of hope. In fact, the process of healing and getting well includes redefining your attitudes and beliefs about IBS so that there is hope. As you'll learn later in this book, hope acts as a powerful biochemical prescription for healing.

As Dr. Simonton discovered, your attitude toward treatment is an important predictor of how you are going to respond to treatment, but it is important to understand that there are other unknown factors in the healing equation. Not every illness can be prevented or cured, and not everyone with IBS responds the same to particular treatments. Sometimes perfectly wonderful people—with wonderful attitudes—respond only minimally to certain treatments. Norman Cousins, in his book *Head First: The Biology of Hope,* says "Not every illness can be overcome, but there is always a margin within which life can be lived with meaning and even with a certain measure of joy, despite illness."

## You Did Not Cause Your Disease

Once you realize that changing your attitudes and beliefs may contribute to your getting well, it is only natural to consider that perhaps your attitudes and beliefs caused your disease. This is not true. Disease and illness are complex matters and there is often no way to know why some people get ill and others don't. Chronic illnesses like IBS are far too complex to simply attribute their development to psychological stress or bad attitudes. You may participate in some activities that predispose you to illness or disease, but you do *not* cause your disease. Do not blame yourself. In this book, we're not looking for explanations for why you became ill with IBS; rather, we're suggesting that changes in attitude, belief and behavior can help you get well again.

Next, let's examine how you can direct the forces of your mind toward healing.

# Chapter 22

## *Forces of the Human Mind*

The doctor has a role beyond the prescription pad to
invoke the patient's own bodily resources for healing.
– Norman Cousins

The body weeps the tears the eyes never shed.
– Robert Bly

---

The attitudes and beliefs you hold represent forces of the human
mind that are no less powerful than a physician's prescription pad.
You can direct your attitudes and beliefs toward creating greater
health in much the same way that you can take a penicillin tablet to
help yourself overcome strep throat. In fact, your positive beliefs and
attitudes are powerful biochemical prescriptions, and, as such, errors
in the choice of attitudes and beliefs you hold are no less devastating
than mistakes in medication or surgery.

---

## Premise 3: Your Attitudes and Beliefs Are No Less Powerful than Medications

Directing your attitudes and beliefs toward creating greater health is
what Elliot Dacher calls "intentional healing." In order to harness the
powerful force of intentional healing, you must first understand the
complex way in which your thoughts, feelings, attitudes and beliefs interact with your body in the creation of illness. For this, let's look at "The
Health Mug."

# The Health Mug

The Health Mug model proposes that you are born with a certain capacity for health and well-being, very much like the open space in a mug (Figure 22.1). When your mug is filled up with too much stuff, it spills over. This overflow results in stress-related medical problems, such as rashes, allergies, headaches, high blood pressure, ulcers, irritable bowel symptoms, migraine, autoimmune diseases and even cancer.

The space in your mug can be divided into three basic categories: things you cannot change, things you can change and things you allow to enter your mug. Let's look at these in detail.

### Things you cannot change

You can't change the things that John Bradshaw calls the "fateful elements"—your genetics, gender, age and family history. You are born into a family with unique genetic codes, belief systems and histories. Bradshaw, author of *Healing the Shame That Binds You,* says, "It is out of our fateful elements we carve out our own identity."

## The Health Mug: Does Your Mug Runneth Over?

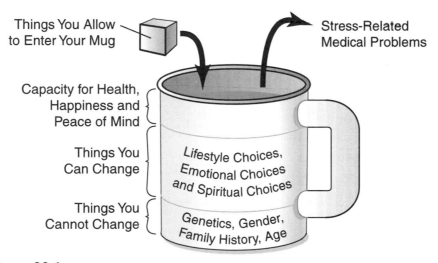

**Figure 22.1**
Reprinted with the permission of Neil F. Neimark, M.D.

By acknowledging these fateful elements—your limitations of genetics, gender, age and family history—you gain power over your powerlessness. If, for example, breast cancer runs in your family, taking extra precautions to detect and prevent it is empowering. If you deny your family history— whether out of fear or ignorance—this genetic predisposition endangers you.

## Things you can change

Certain elements in your mug are the result of the choices you make. These are the MindBodySpirit modifying factors that you were introduced to in Chapter 9. They include lifestyle choices, emotional choices and spiritual choices.

1. *Lifestyle choices:* poor diet, workaholism, lack of exercise, high stress, smoking, lack of play/recreation and inadequate preventive care, such as not having regular mammograms, PAP smears, prostate checks and colon screens.
2. *Emotional choices:* unresolved anger, grief, resentment, excessive fear or worry, frustration, guilt, being a victim (helplessness), self-criticism, lack of loving relationships, toxic shame, blaming others, blaming yourself, denial and doubt. These emotional choices are what Elisabeth Kubler-Ross, author of *On Death and Dying,* calls "unfinished business."
3. *Spiritual choices:* deep sense of unworthiness, low self-esteem, toxic shame (the feeling that you're not loved for who you are), a sense of isolation, lack of direction, lack of higher purpose, lack of meaning, lack of an inner life and lack of a higher power.

## Things you allow to enter your mug

In addition to the internal elements that fill up your mug, your health is always being threatened by outside forces that include viruses, bacteria, environmental pollutants and psychosocial stressors. These triggers/stressors act like ice cubes thrown into your mug, taking up valuable space as they melt. Some of these outside forces include other people's anger, other people's guilt, other people's criticism, other people's abusiveness, environmental noise, toxic work situations, unsupportive friends, unsafe sex, excessive traffic jams and unrealistic expectations. If you add too many of these stressful ice cubes, your mug will overflow, resulting in stress-related illness.

## The space left over

The space left in your mug (after room has been taken up by all of the "things" in your mug) represents your capacity for health, happiness and peace of mind. The Health Mug shows that the maintenance of health is a remarkable balancing act. Certain elements inside your mug cannot change. Other elements are constantly in flux and vary in intensity—like your level of anger, stress, sadness, frustration and disappointment. Lastly, external forces constantly threaten your health. The space left in your mug—your capacity for health, happiness and peace of mind—varies from moment to moment. Step 2 described the neurobiology of allostasis, which is the dynamic process of maintaining internal balance (homeostasis)—the effort that your MindBodySpirit Connection makes on behalf of your health. When you empty your mug and decrease your allostatic load and the bad stress response, you increase your healing capacity. This capacity represents not only your ability to reduce and eliminate symptoms and fight off disease, but also your ability to enjoy life, to play and to live well. The space created as you empty your mug holds your joys, allowing you to drink life's sweet nectar and celebrate your aliveness.

# Illness as Wakeup Call

Achieving and maintaining health requires us to ask what is filling up our mugs. Asking this question *before* your mug is overflowing enables you to minimize or prevent stress-related illness. Rachel Naomi Remen, M.D., director of the Commonweal Cancer Program in northern California, states that illness has become a form of western meditation. She says, "Illness awakens in people a need to understand the deeper issues that underlie daily life. Illness is like a wakeup call."

For most people, it is only after they become ill that they examine what's filling up their mug. When you look deep inside, you discover that much of the "stuff" filling up your mug is related to your attitudes and beliefs. At the spiritual level, your feelings of shame, unworthiness, isolation and low self-esteem often stem from erroneous beliefs about yourself and your sense of belonging to the world. At the emotional level, unexpressed anger, deeply held resentments, sadness and grief reflect self-limiting beliefs about the world you live in and the nature of your relationships in life.

Emotionally, the process of finishing your unfinished business involves going through the stages of grief, which always lead to anger, sadness and tears. These tears represent your anger, hurt, disappointment and pain that things didn't turn out the way you had hoped. Shedding tears represents letting go and saying goodbye, necessary steps in order to make room for newness and hope. Failing to release these tears places you at risk for overflow, excess allostatic load and the creation of stress-related illness with worsening of your IBS. Poet and author Robert Bly says, "The body weeps the tears the eyes never shed." What you fail to feel or grieve in your emotional life may manifest as illness in your body.

## Putting Words to Your Feelings

You drain unresolved emotions from your mug by putting words to your feelings—by speaking to friends, sharing in a support group or expressing yourself through art, music, poetry or journaling. Whatever means you use, putting words to your feelings is vital for healing. It increases the capacity of your mug to hold health, happiness and peace of mind. Expressing painful feelings results in tears, sadness, anger and fear. Research shows that emotional tears differ in composition from tears produced by chemical irritants. Emotional tears remove toxins from the body.

F.I. Fawzy and N.W. Fawzy (*Archives of General Psychiatry,* 1993;Sept.; 50(9);681–9) studied patients in the early stages of malignant melanoma and found that expressing anger at having the disease had a positive, stimulating effect on the immune system, increasing natural killer cell activity. Repressed anger, not expressed anger, damages your body and psyche. There are appropriate and inappropriate ways to express your anger, but repression is rarely—if ever—the answer.

Many of your unresolved emotions were acquired in childhood. You learned that your anger or your fear was unacceptable. But as a child, you didn't have the words—or the freedom—to express yourself, so the anger and fear stayed locked inside your body. This is what John Bradshaw calls "preverbal powerlessness." When you put adult words to your needs and feelings, you break out of your preverbal powerlessness. You reclaim your power and increase your capacity for physical and emotional joy. Expressing your feelings may be frightening and threatening, but it is also healing.

# Guard Your Mug

Because your health is always being threatened by outside forces, you must be cautious about what you let into your mug. If other people's anger or guilt enters your mug, it plops in with a big splash, raising the level of your mug. If your mug is already full, that other person's anger or guilt causes your mug to overflow into a stress-related illness. People love to throw their stuff into your mug. The way that you can prevent this from happening is by setting boundaries. Setting appropriate boundaries is like standing guard at the entrance to your mug.

Appropriate physical, emotional and spiritual boundaries protect you and heal you in two main ways: (1) by preventing you from spending precious time, energy and worry taking care of things that are not your responsibility and (2) by helping you recognize those things that are your responsibility. In studies on stress and immune function, UCLA psychiatrist and researcher George Solomon, M.D., found that the best correlation with strong immune function was the ability to say "no" to a request for a favor. Setting clear limits and boundaries reduces unnecessary stress and says, "I value myself. I value my needs. I value who I am and what I believe." Setting limits gives your body a "live" message.

## Setting boundaries

There is always a spirited response when people hear about Dr. Solomon's study. The fact that saying "no" to a request for a favor can have such powerful implications for your immune system fascinates us. We all struggle with boundaries. Saying "no" to people you love sometimes feels selfish and unkind. Yet establishing healthy boundaries is anything but unkind—in fact, it is one of the kindest steps you can take toward achieving true intimacy with those you love.

Saying "yes" when you really want to say "no" is dishonest with yourself and others. It leads to resentment—and resentment eventually comes out, either toward others or toward your own body, perhaps as the symptoms of IBS. Setting healthy boundaries does not mean you always say "no," but it does mean that your "yes" really means "yes." This honesty allows you to reach out, be kind and help others who really need your help—while it protects you from the burdensome weight of helping others who are too lazy or irresponsible to help themselves.

An excellent definition of boundaries is given by Dr. Henry Cloud and Dr. John Townsend in their insightful and powerful book, *Boundaries: When to Say YES, When to Say NO, to Take Control of Your Life*. They say, "A boundary is a personal property line that marks those things for which you are responsible. In other words, boundaries define who you are and who you are not." Physical boundaries determine who may touch you and when. Mental boundaries define what you think and believe. Emotional boundaries give you space to deal with your own feelings and disengage from or protect yourself from hurtful or manipulative feelings of others.

When you set appropriate boundaries, you say "no" to other peoples' anger, unrealistic expectations, hurtfulness, demands, guilt and shame. You become the master of your destiny—freeing yourself from the bondage of needing other peoples' approval. We all want the good will and best wishes of others, but—as adults—we do not need the approval of others to be happy.

Learn more about boundaries.

# Chemical Thoughts, Chemical Feelings

What you say to yourself when dealing with other people's or your own issues is important because thoughts and feelings are chemical. The thoughts you speak to yourself and the feelings you experience are translated through the three MindBodySpirit communication systems (CNS, CMS and ANS) into neurosignatures: unique patterns of nerve cell firing and chemical release (Chapter 3). These chemical messenger molecules carry your thoughts and feelings throughout your body. The implications of this are profound because nearly every cell in your body has receptor sites for these chemical messenger molecules of thought and emotion. These receptor sites "listen" to and physically record the conversations you have with yourself. If you always put others first, what are you really saying to yourself? "I am worth less than you." I am "worthless." When your body hears this type of message, there are physical, cellular and immune consequences.

# Same Insult, Different Responses

Now that you understand the many dynamic elements within your health mug, you can see that different people may respond quite differently to the same disease-causing agent. Imagine that an ice cube in the form of bacteria plops into your Health Mug. If your mug is already full, the bacteria cause your mug to overflow, causing a respiratory infection. However, if your mug has room in it, that same ice cube does not result in overflow and you do not get sick! Thus, two different people exposed to the same bacteria can have very different responses; one becomes ill, while the other stays well. Learn more about <u>stress and infections</u>.

When you realize the multitude of things that can fill up your mug, you understand the complexity of how allostatic load and the bad stress response interact with your body. This complexity is reflected in the words of William Osler, M.D., the first chief of medicine at Johns Hopkins University, who said, "It is much more important to know what sort of patient has the disease than what sort of disease the patient has."

In the next chapter, you will discover the mechanisms for healing: your inner pharmacy and the power of your positive beliefs to create remarkable physical and biochemical changes in your mind, body and spirit.

# Chapter 23

## *Mechanisms for Healing*

[I] further proclaimed that the body was God's drugstore and had
in it all liquids, drugs, lubricating oils, opiates, acids and anti-acids,
and every sort of drug which the wisdom of God thought necessary
for human happiness and health.

– Andrew Taylor Still

---

You have an inner pharmacy that produces an endless array of neurotransmitters, neuropeptides, hormones, antibodies and chemical
agents that fight off disease, improve immunity, relieve pain and
restore health and balance to your physiology and biochemistry. Your
inner pharmacy is an important tool in the treatment of your IBS.

---

## Positive Belief and the Placebo Response

Scientists and healers have long known about the incredible power of
positive belief and expectancy. You have already learned the vital role that
positive attitudes and beliefs play in achieving greater health and healing
for your IBS. *What you may not know is that the power of positive belief is
the placebo response.* Most people have heard of the placebo response and
understand it to be a sugar pill or inert element that is given to people in
order to test the efficacy of new drugs or in order to "treat" people who
worry too much when there is really nothing wrong with them! Although
treatment with placebo is not intentionally done in modern day practice,
it is of interest that many times you can create a "placebo response" without the "placebo." In these cases, your belief in the doctor or caregiver
acts as the placebo. You don't need to swallow a "sugar pill" to obtain the
benefits of positive belief (placebo). In order to better understand the

remarkable self-healing abilities available to you through the power of positive belief, let's first start with a definition.

Howard Brody, M.D., Ph.D., and author of *The Placebo Response,* says, "The placebo response is a change in the body that occurs as the result of the symbolic significance which one attributes to an event or object in the healing environment." This definition expands the scope of the placebo response beyond the sugar pill and, as you will see, shows how "belief in something," along with a change in the symbolic meaning of an event, can have positive health benefits.

In the early stages of studying the placebo response, studies showed that about one-third of patients benefited from placebos. That is, when you gave one group of patients the active drug and another group of patients the placebo, approximately 33% of those patients who received the placebo got better. This, in itself, is remarkable. However, Roberts and colleagues (*Clinical Psychology Review,* 1993; 13:375–91) showed that in the settings of heightened expectancy, the placebo response could rise to an average rate of 70% improvement! In his book *Timeless Healing,* Herbert Benson, M.D., concurs with this opinion and cites three key factors that increase the ability of the placebo response to effect positive health changes. Let's take a look at them.

# Increasing the Healing Power of Positive Belief

Self-healing through the power of positive belief is increased by three key factors. The first factor is belief and expectancy on the part of the patient. This occurs when the patient has a strong belief in the positive benefits of the treatment (whether it be a drug, procedure or other treatment). The second factor is belief and expectancy on the part of the caregiver. This occurs when the doctor or caregiver has a strong belief in the positive benefits of the treatment. The third factor is belief and expectancy generated by the relationship between the caregiver and the patient. When the patient and the doctor believe and trust in one another, self-healing is heightened.

By utilizing these three factors, you can increase and augment the healing power of your beliefs. You can also see why it is so important to have a doctor you trust and a treatment plan you have faith in.

# The Nocebo Response

The power of belief, when positive in influence, is called the placebo response. The power of belief, when negative in influence, is called the nocebo response. Negative expectations can create negative outcomes. For example, many patients believe they will get the flu every December, and—like clockwork—when December comes around, they get the flu. Remember, the power of belief is neutral, like a knife. When used by a surgeon, a knife can save a life. When used by a thug, it can destroy a life. Your beliefs are like a knife. You can use them to heal or to harm.

# How the Placebo Response Works

In trying to understand the different ways in which the placebo response works, Dr. Brody describes three complementary models that work together to create positive health changes (*Journal of Family Practice,* 2000;49:649–654). These are the Meaning Model, the Expectancy Model and the Conditioning Model.

> 1. *The Meaning Model* is active when a change in the meaning you assign to an illness or to a form of treatment creates a positive health benefit.
> 2. *The Expectancy Model* is active when a change in what you expect or anticipate creates a positive health benefit.
> 3. *The Conditioning Model* is active when repeated past experiences create a pattern of bodily change that may be replicated in the present.

Before we discuss each model in more detail, let's first discuss the concept of the "inner pharmacy."

# Your Body's Inner Pharmacy

Dr. Brody's concept of an "inner pharmacy" explains how all three models of the placebo response stimulate the healing power of positive belief. The inner pharmacy represents your body's ability to produce an endless array of neuropeptides, neurotransmitters, hormones, antibodies and chemical agents to fight off disease, improve immunity, increase energy, relieve pain and restore health and balance to your physiology and biochemistry. The inner pharmacy is not confined to any particular anatomic location. The brain and central nervous system manufacture a wide variety of neuro-chemicals, but circulating white cells can produce them as well.

Through the three mechanisms already mentioned (changes in meaning, expectancy and conditioning), your mind (or body) sends a prescription to your inner pharmacy. When this message (prescription) is received by your inner pharmacist, the appropriate chemical molecules are dispensed into your bloodstream and body tissues.

In this respect, you and your doctor both have prescription writing privileges. So, like a doctor, you must learn to use your prescribing privi-leges wisely. Every thought, feeling, attitude and belief you have has the potential to write a prescription to your inner pharmacy through the CNS, CMS and ANS. You can now appreciate how vital it is that you reach within to mobilize your own internal resources for healing in addi-tion to following your doctor's prescribed treatments.

Now, let's discuss in detail the three models for how the power of belief works. As you learn about each model, keep in mind that each model repre-sents a different way in which a prescription is sent to your inner pharmacy.

# The Meaning Model

The meaning model states that any positive change in the meaning you assign to an event, treatment or illness creates positive health benefits for you. The meaning model basically asks, "How does what I believe about my illness—its meaning to me—affect my inner pharmacy?" Positive change in the meaning of an illness occurs when (1) you feel listened to and receive a clear and satisfactory explanation of your illness; (2) you feel the care and concern of those around you; and (3) you feel an enhanced sense of mastery and control over your symptoms.

The meaning model reveals how powerful your mind can be in helping you control your IBS. For example, when you learn a new relaxation technique that gives you an enhanced sense of mastery over your symptoms, you not only benefit by improved relaxation, but the enhanced mastery sends a "change in meaning" message to your inner pharmacy. The pharmacy then dispenses appropriate neurochemicals that induce a further sense of calm and symptom relief.

Another important way to enhance your sense of mastery over IBS is by taking the time to listen to your body in an attempt to understand why and what brings you greater health and well-being. You have a tremendous inner wisdom that no one else does about your own unique bodily needs. It is vital that you be proactive in discovering things that you can do, at least some of the time, to help alleviate or minimize your troublesome IBS symptoms. Don't over-rely on your doctor to supply every treatment option. Never underestimate your own intuitive ability to find changes in diet, attitude or spirituality that can dramatically alter your health for the better. Your doctor is your coach, and can advise you, but you must be out there practicing your game.

The meaning model also relates to what you already learned about "story work" or "narrative about illness." Consciously or unconsciously, you attach meaning to events and situations in your life by constructing a narrative or story about different events. Since many of the meanings attached to illness are filled with pain, negativity and hurt, when you have a chance to rewrite those narratives (through journaling or through "talking things out"), you can effect a change in meaning that has a positive influence on your health and healing.

You are probably unaware that many of the meanings you have attached to your IBS were unconsciously chosen by you. Because of this, your story may include unnecessarily painful outcome scenarios. It is important to bring the invisible stories (and meanings) about your IBS into the visible world of conscious awareness, so that you can begin to rewrite your stories.

What negative meanings have you attached to your story about IBS? Do you have any guilt feelings? Any stories of anger and frustration? Any sadness or goodbye stories that relate to your IBS? The stories you create become part of the very fabric of your cellular and biochemical memory. Therefore, it is important to construct alternative stories or different endings to your stories. Use your imagination to create happier, more peaceful endings to your story.

Dr. Brody says that at the beginning of treatment, patients often see only two possible stories: a future in which their pain magically disappears completely or one in which they suffer forever. With proper support, insight and exploration, you can rewrite your story so that it includes "the possibility of feeling less pain and achieving important life goals despite never being completely cured."

# The Expectancy Model

This model teaches that if you expect to improve after you receive a certain medicine or treatment, there's a good chance that you will improve— even if the improvement cannot be explained by any of the chemical components in the medication or treatment. In this model, bodily changes occur in relationship to the degree that you expect them to. As in all placebo responses, the bodily effect can be beneficial or harmful depending on what your expectations are. The expectancy model basically asks, "How does what I think is going to happen in the future affect my inner pharmacy?" What you expect to occur sends a clear prescription to your inner pharmacy, which then works toward creating the expected bodily effect. What are the implications for you and your IBS? What do you expect regarding the various treatments prescribed for your illness? How can you begin to change your expectations, or alter them in a way that brings you the positive benefits of your inner pharmacy?

Learn more about the expectancy model.

## Negative expectancy: The nocebo response

No study of the power of positive belief is complete without looking at the power of negative beliefs (the nocebo response). Just as positive expectancy can generate health and healing, so negative beliefs or negative expectancy—as you just learned—can have a detrimental or even catastrophic effect on your health and healing.

One of the most dramatic illustrations of the power of negative beliefs is a study by J.W. Fielding at the Department of Surgery, Queen Elizabeth Hospital, Birmingham, England (*World Journal of Surgery*, 1983; 390–399). In this study, 411 patients were told to expect hair loss from a chemotherapy agent about to be administered. Thirty percent of these patients unknowingly received a placebo instead of the chemotherapy agent. This "placebo" group lost their hair even though the pills they took contained no active medication.

Learn more about <u>negative expectancy</u>.

## The Conditioning Model

In this model, bodily changes occur when you are exposed to a stimulus that has been linked in the past to positive or negative health changes. The conditioning model basically asks, "How does what has happened to me in the past affect my inner pharmacy?"

A common example of this occurs when a patient walks out in the rain barefoot and a few days later coincidentally comes down with a severe cold. Several weeks later, the same patient goes out in the rain barefoot and catches a cold again. Now, every time this patient goes out in the rain barefoot, he becomes ill. The effect is probably augmented by memories of his mother calling, "Don't go out in the rain barefoot. You'll catch a cold!" The patient has now become "conditioned to illness" when walking barefoot in the rain. In other words, a state of negative bodily health has been linked to a stimulus (walking barefoot in the rain). Though this example is simplified, many new treatments have been created to help people heal from proper "conditioning" using the placebo response.

The conditioning model holds great promise in helping patients. You may wonder how the conditioning model is related to the power of positive belief, because by definition, the conditioning model does not require the patient to believe the treatment will work in order to see the positive effect. Scientists know this because many conditioning experiments have been done in laboratory animals (who do not "believe" in the treatment) and they still find the same positive health benefits. How then is the conditioning model related to the power of positive belief?

In the conditioning model, the *body* is made to "believe" that the substance it is receiving or exposed to is the same as a drug. Remember that every one of your body cells has a memory of past events. Because initially, a drug is administered together with a stimulus, the body memory cannot distinguish the effect of one from the other. Therefore, when the body receives the stimulus, it "believes" (through cellular memory) that the drug is also present.

Learn more about the <u>conditioning model</u>.

Let's now move on to Step 5, where you will learn how to take an active and responsible role in managing your IBS by learning how to care for your body.

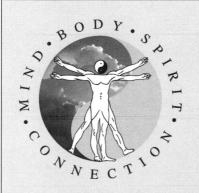

The possibilities for healing through a greater understanding of the power of belief are very promising. You will experience new and unexpected opportunities for health and healing if you maintain a positive attitude about your life by:

- Expressing your honest feelings
- Constructing healthier narratives about your IBS
- Cultivating positive attitudes and beliefs
- Eliminating negative attitudes and beliefs about your IBS

You will find new opportunities in the realms of mind, body and spirit.

# STEP 5

## CARING FOR YOUR BODY

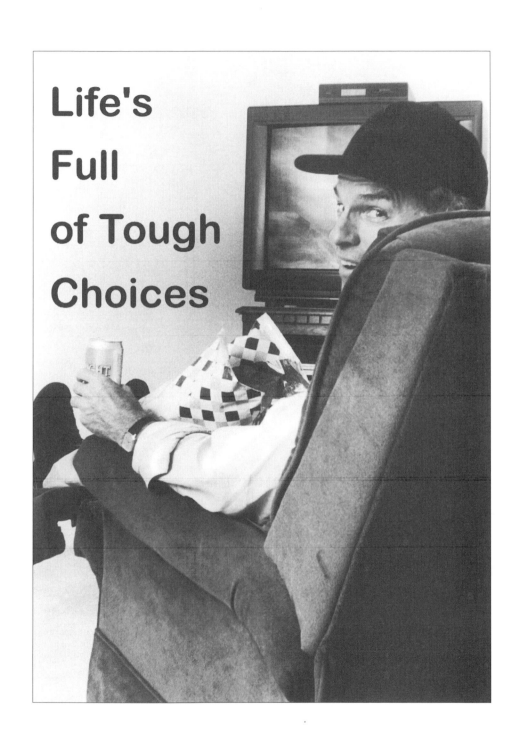

# Chapter 24
## *Healing: Your Responsibility*

**Work with your doctor, and with unconventional practitioners
if you so choose, to learn self-care habits. . . . I consider self-care
anything an individual can do, independent of doctors or healers,
to enhance his or her health.**
— *Timeless Healing: The Power and Biology of Belief*
Herbert Benson, M.D. (with Marg Stark)

You can heal. *You are the only one who can do it.* Your ability to heal
comes through understanding the MindBodySpirit Connection,
accepting responsibility for your health, reducing your allostatic
load and making a commitment to self-care.

## Understanding the MindBodySpirit Connection

"Knowledge is power," and you have both when you understand the
MindBodySpirit Connection. You know that mind, body and spirit are
inseparably linked. Your thoughts, feelings, attitudes and beliefs are transmitted throughout your body by the three MindBodySpirit communication systems (CNS, CMS and ANS), which are similar to the different
sections of instruments in an orchestra. The musical conductor of these
three systems is the brain neuromatrix, where mind, body and spirit meet.
With each and every event, thought and feeling, your brain neuromatrix
(the conductor) signals the three MindBodySpirit communication systems
to "play" a neurosignature (a unique pattern of nerve cell firing and chemical release) that sets the tone for how you feel physically, mentally and
spiritually.

You now understand that to say something is "all in your head" no longer makes sense, because what is "in your head" is also "in your body." Your mind (thoughts, feelings, attitudes and beliefs) is not confined to your brain, but circulates to—and permeates within—every cell in your body.

You have a new and positive language: MindBodySpirit medicine and healing. You understand your IBS and other functional symptoms and syndromes through the interaction of the MindBodySpirit Connection with heredity and the environment. You can reduce your allostatic load.

# Taking Responsibility

The model of interaction between patient and doctor is changing. You, the patient, must now assume responsibility for your health in partnership with your doctor. To do so, you must have the information and knowledge, because they are as important—often more important—than medication. Information and knowledge lead to healing.

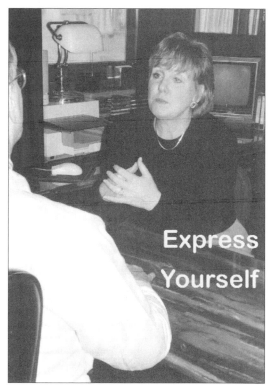

Partner with Your Doctor

Healing your IBS requires attention directed to your whole being: mind, body and spirit. Remember, all forms of treatment require you to *reach out* for the best that medical science has to offer and to *reach in* to mobilize your own internal resources for healing. Treatment of IBS directed to the body and gut alone—without addressing the mind and spirit—may be well intentioned, but is unlikely to lead to enduring healing.

## Taking Control

A sense of mastery or control is a vital pathway to your healing system, and your commitment and decision to take control are just as important as the details of your strategy. Norman Cousins wrote, "In general, anything that restores a sense of control to a patient can be a profound aid to a physician in treating serious illness. That sense of control is more than a mere mood or attitude and may well be a vital pathway between the brain, the endocrine system and the immune system. The assumed possibility is that it may serve as the basis for what may well be a profound advance in the knowledge of how to confront the challenge of serious illness" (*Head First: The Biology of Hope*).

This sense of control is achieved by taking small steps in the direction of your goals. Don't be a "weekend warrior" and try to get fit in one weekend. Take small steps. Your perseverance and determination are as critical to mastery as lifting weights are to building big biceps. Master musicians first practice their routine and boring scales day in and day out, before they can play the masterpieces. Master healers must first practice the simple principles of health and wellness day in and day out, before they can master wellness.

## Putting IBS to Work for You

As we said in the Introduction, "You can 'use' IBS to change your life and health." You can turn the negative of your illness into the positive of health. *You are the only one who can do it. It takes commitment and change, but not only can you heal from IBS, you can also be healthier than you have ever been before.* Remember that with each small step of self-care you build a stronger, healthier and more joyous body—a beautiful home for your mind and spirit to dwell in.

There is a story of an elderly carpenter who was about to retire after a long and satisfying career. His employer—disappointed at the timing of his retirement—asked him one last favor: to build one more house before he retired. The carpenter—feeling obligated to his long-time employer—

begrudgingly agreed. As he began his work, it was clear that his heart was not in the job. He used inferior materials, shoddy worksmanship, cut corners and did not live up to his usual high standards of craftsmanship. When the job was complete, the employer came out to inspect the house, and as he approached the carpenter, he handed him the keys to the house, saying, "This is my gift to you. I wanted to provide you with one final thanks for all the good work and kindness you have shown me over the years."

So it is with the house called our body. We can cut corners, use inferior materials and shoddy worksmanship, but this is our house, the one we must live in, the gift we were all given.

In the next chapter, you will learn about the importance of sleep in IBS.

# Chapter 25
## *Sleep*

O sleep, O gentle sleep,
Nature's soft nurse.
– *Henry IV*
Shakespeare

---

Many people who are otherwise healthy and most patients with IBS and other functional syndromes have trouble sleeping. Sleep disturbance contributes to IBS symptom severity and chronicity by setting up an unhealthy vicious cycle. Poor sleep contributes to your allostatic load. Obtaining proper sleep can help you heal from IBS.

---

Approximately one-third of adult Americans complain about sleeping trouble. The National Commission on Sleep Disorders reported in 1992 that about 40 million Americans suffer from sleep-wake disorders, that many are undiagnosed and untreated and that only one in five people goes to see a doctor about the problem. The hectic pace of our lives also cuts into sleep time, and poor lifestyle choices contribute to poor sleep.

## IBS Consequences of Poor Sleep

Most patients with IBS and other functional syndromes report poor sleep. IBS and sleep disturbance are a vicious cycle. The bad stress response of allostatic load leads to abdominal pain and bowel disturbance, alterations of the mind/brain, emotional distress, increased vigilance and symptoms of anxiety and depression. The disturbance of sleep increases gut and bodily sensitivity, which increases symptoms and distress. Scientific studies have shown that the symptoms of IBS and fibromyalgia can be produced in otherwise healthy adults by sleep deprivation. Poor and inadequate sleep contribute to allostatic load.

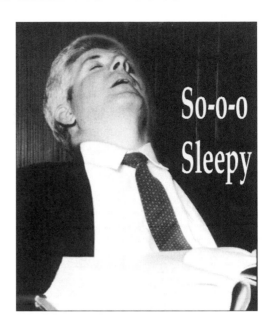

## The Neurobiology of Sleep Disturbance

Stage 4 sleep is the phase of sleep called deep sleep. It is also called non-rapid eye movement (nREM) sleep. Most patients with IBS and other functional syndromes, such as fibromyalgia, have abnormalities of Stage 4 sleep that contribute to awakening in the morning feeling tired and unrefreshed.

Another phase of sleep is called rapid eye movement sleep (REM), which is associated with dreaming, arousal, altered activity of the autonomic nervous system and altered colon function. Increased REM sleep occurs in some patients with IBS and other functional syndromes.

## Getting Better Sleep

Table 25.1 lists our recommendations for improving your sleep.

| Table 25.1 |
| :-- |
| ### Approach to Better Sleep |
| General |
| • Relax for at least one hour before going to bed. |
| • Allow the mind and body to relax (for example, by meditating). |
| • Go to bed only when sleepy. |
| • Get out of bed if you are unable to sleep. |
| *(continued on next page)* |

Table 25.1 *(continued from previous page)*
- Keep a regular sleep schedule.
- Reserve the bed and bedroom for sleep and sex.
- Try not to sleep during the day. However, short naps (from 10 to 30 minutes) may be helpful energy boosters for many people and do not usually interfere with nighttime sleep.
- Avoid heavy meals before bedtime.
- Avoid caffeine and alcohol, particularly in the evening.
- Get regular exercise, but avoid it just before bedtime (Chapters 29 and 30).

Stress management and relaxation techniques (Chapter 34)

Cognitive behavioral therapy (Chapter 35)

Medication (Chapter 18)

"Natural" remedies (Chapter 18)

Sleep study in the laboratory

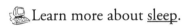Learn more about <u>sleep</u>.

In the next chapter, we'll discuss the fundamentals of a healthy diet.

# Chapter 26

## *Healthy Diet*

Eat your fruits and vegetables.
– Your Mother

A poor diet contributes to your allostatic load. Committing to a healthy diet is an important step in taking control of—and responsibility for—your health and recovery from IBS. Furthermore, your life depends upon it.

In Step 3, you reviewed specific dietary issues regarding IBS, but eating a healthy diet is most important. Scientific studies show that over 300,000 people die every year as a result of diseases related to poor diet and inadequate physical activity. A healthy diet reduces the risk of developing heart disease, high blood pressure, high cholesterol, some forms of cancer, diabetes, stroke and osteoporosis by reducing allostatic load. These are the leading causes of death and disability among Americans today. Because we have control over our diet and exercise, these major killers have been termed "diseases of choice, not chance."

## Dietary Confusion

Most people are confused about what constitutes a healthy diet as well as how to lose and maintain weight. There are many popular diets available, particularly for achieving weight loss, and they often give conflicting advice. For example, cardiologist Robert Atkins recommends a high-protein, low carbohydrate regimen that includes considerable saturated fat. Other popular low carbohydrate diets include *The Carbohydrate*

*Addict's Diet, Protein Power, Sugar Busters!, The Zone* and *Get Skinny on Fabulous Foods.* By contrast, Dean Ornish, M.D.—an outspoken critic of low carbohydrate diets—advocates an ultra-low fat vegetarian diet. Cyndi Thompson, a spokeswoman for the American Dietetic Association and a nutrition expert at the University of Arizona, says, "We have millions of dollars being spent on these diets, and everyone is throwing rocks at each other over what is the best diet." The United States Department of Agriculture is conducting scientific studies of popular diets—such as the Atkins and Ornish regimens—at their nutrition research center at the University of California, Davis.

Learn more about <u>healthy eating</u>.

# Eating Rules

Whenever possible, try to select fresh foods and unprocessed foods. Foods prepared by others before they get to our households are more likely to have added salt, sugar, saturated fats, preservatives and artificial coloring. Furthermore, fiber and nutritional content decrease with the increased processing required to give foods a longer shelf life.

Eat in moderation and only when you're hungry and while you are in a relaxed, unhurried atmosphere. Take the time to chew food properly and enjoy the sensations. This nourishes not only your body but also your mind and spirit. Chewing properly and eating slowly are vital to healthy digestion. This alone may relieve many of your uncomfortable IBS symptoms. In addition, eating more frequent, smaller meals throughout the day may result in less discomfort than eating one or two larger meals.

# Dietary Guidelines for Americans

The Dietary Guidelines for Americans (DGA) are issued jointly by the U.S. Department of Agriculture and the Department of Health and Human Services every five years. They are available from the U.S.

Department of Agriculture as a 44-page booklet or on the Internet. Learn more about <u>DGA</u>.

The ten recommendations of the DGA 2000 are listed below. After them, specific components of nutritional health are discussed.

1. **Aim for a healthy weight.** Body mass should not exceed 25 kg/m$^2$ and waist measurement should be less than 35 inches for women and 40 inches for men (Chapter 28).

2. **Be physically active each day.** Adults should get 30 minutes of moderate exercise each day; children should get 60 minutes (Chapters 29 and 30).

3. **Let the food pyramid guide your food choices.** Per day, most people need nine servings of bread, cereal, rice and pasta; four of vegetables; three of fruit; two or three of dairy; and two of meat, fish or poultry.

4. **Choose a variety of grains daily, especially whole grains.** Of the six to nine servings a day, at least three should be whole grains.

5. **Choose a variety of fruits and vegetables daily.** The new guidelines specifically call attention to eating fruits and vegetables; only 17 percent of Americans eat the recommended amount of fruit and only 30 percent eat the recommended amount of vegetables per day.

6. **Keep food safe to eat.** Raw and uncooked foods should be kept separate. Foods can become contaminated at cooking temperatures below 140°F and refrigeration temperatures above 40°F.

7. **Choose a diet low in saturated fat and cholesterol and moderate in total fat.** No more than 30 percent of calories should be from fat, with 10 percent from saturated fats and 20 percent from unsaturated fats.

8. **Choose beverages and foods with less sugar.** Soft drinks are the leading source of added sugar in the American diet.

9. **Choose and prepare foods with less salt.** Use herbs and seasonings instead.

10. **If you drink alcoholic beverages, do so in moderation.** The cardiovascular benefit of one drink a day is proven only in women over age 55 and men over age 45.

# Carbohydrates

Carbohydrates serve as the body's main source of calories (energy) and should comprise 50 to 60 percent of your total caloric intake. Most of your carbohydrates should be eaten as beans, vegetables, fruits and whole grains.

By definition, a whole grain food has at least 51 percent whole grain by weight. However, most Americans do not understand what whole-grain foods are. Unlike refined grains, whole-grains have considerably more fiber and are rich in nutrients, antioxidants and cancer preventive substances. A whole grain contains all three major parts of the grain: bran (outer layer), endosperm (large middle portion) and germ (core). Processing removes bran.

Examples of whole grains include wild rice, brown rice (including instant), popcorn, bulgur wheat, whole wheat kernels, oats and oatmeal, barley (including pearled barley), buckwheat, kasha, cracked wheat, quinoa (pronounced *keen-wa*) and amaranth. Examples of grains that are not whole grains are white rice, cornmeal and whole kernel corn (which is a vegetable).

Breakfast cereals should indicate whether they are whole grain products. Look for the words "whole-grain" or "rich in whole-grain." Examples of cereals that are more than 90 percent whole-grain include Cheerios, regular oatmeal, shredded wheat and Wheaties. All-bran cereals are an exception. Technically, they are not whole-grain, but they are so loaded with bran that they have the value of whole-grain.

Breads and crackers require a careful review of labels. The first ingredient should have the word *whole* in it, such as whole-wheat (another name is graham flour), whole oats, whole rye flour and whole barley. Search for whole-wheat crackers (for example, Triscuits), whole-wheat tortillas, whole grain bagels, couscous and whole wheat pasta.

# Fat

There are two main types of fat: (1) saturated fat, which is solid at room temperature and (2) unsaturated fat, which is liquid at room temperature. In general, saturated fat comes from animal products and carries the greatest health risk, while unsaturated fat comes from vegetable sources. Limit fat intake to 30 percent or less of total calories consumed. In other words, on a 2,000 calorie per day diet, 600 calories or about 67 grams should come from fat. Most fat should be in the form of monounsaturated oils and fats and oils rich in omega-3 essential fatty acids, which are discussed below.

## Saturated fat

Keep your consumption of saturated fats low. The more saturated fat you consume, the greater your risk of developing high cholesterol, heart attack, stroke, circulation problems and certain types of cancer (like colon cancer). Furthermore, there are more calories in each gram of saturated fat (9 calories) than there are in each gram of protein (4 calories) or carbohydrate (4 calories). If you eat fatty foods, you are more likely to have a weight problem. Limit saturated fat intake by eating fewer fried foods (most fast foods), butter, cream, cheese, other full-fat dairy products, unskinned chicken, fatty meats and products made with palm and coconut oil.

## Trans-fatty acids (trans-fats) (hydrogenated fat)

*Trans*-fatty acids are a harmful type of manufactured fat produced from unsaturated vegetable oils through a process called hydrogenation. Trans-fatty acids lead to higher elevations of blood fats and to more blood vessel and heart disease than saturated fats (*New England Journal of Medicine,* 1999;340:1994–1997). Pay careful attention to foods like crackers, baked goods, margarine and other prepared foods with the words "hydrogenated" or "partially hydrogenated" listed in the ingredients. Many fast foods—like doughnuts and french fries—contain high levels of trans-fatty acids.

### Polyunsaturated fats

These are called omega-6 vegetable fatty acids. Reduce your consumption of polyunsaturated vegetable oils, which include safflower, sunflower, sesame, corn, soy, cottonseed and products that are made from them.

### "Good fats"

*Monounsaturated fat.*   Olive oil—a monounsaturated omega-9 fat—is better for your body than either saturated or polyunsaturated fat. Cultures that rely upon olive oil as their main dietary source of fat have lower rates of both heart disease and cancer than Americans do, even though their total fat intake is not lower. Olive oil is still fat, and each gram contains 9 calories, so don't overdo it. Other sources of monounsaturated fats include cashews, pistachios and macadamias.

*Omega-3 fatty acids.*   Omega-3 fatty acids are beneficial to health but cannot be manufactured by the body. They inhibit the clotting tendency of the blood, reduce the risk of heart attack and lower cholesterol and triglycerides. They also have beneficial effects on the brain and mental health. Omega-3 fatty acids modify the production of hormones that control tissue growth and repair, thereby reducing excessive inflammation and promoting wound healing. Sources include oily fish from cold, northern waters (kippers, herring, mackerel, salmon and sardines). Non-fish sources include flax seed, walnuts, pumpkin seeds, soy and eggs from free-range chickens or which are "fortified" with omega-3 fatty acids.

# Cholesterol

Cholesterol from foods has only a slight influence on blood cholesterol and fats compared to the effects of saturated fat and trans-fatty acids. Nonetheless, we still recommend that you consider limiting your cholesterol intake to less than 300 mg per day.

# Protein

Protein should comprise 10 to 20 percent of total caloric intake. On a 2000 calorie per day diet, this would be 50 to 100 grams. Eat more vegetable protein, especially from beans, soybeans and nuts, and eat less animal protein, with the exception of fish and reduced-fat dairy products. Recommended protein intake also depends upon your level of activity and may need to be increased if you exercise more.

# Fiber

The optimal diet should include 20–35 grams of fiber per day. You may need to use a fiber supplement to achieve this amount of fiber. Refer to Chapter 17 for a more detailed discussion.

# Fluid

Drink at least six to eight glasses of fluid per day. Adequate fluid intake is particularly important when taking fiber supplements.

# Soy

In October of 1999, the U.S. Food and Drug Administration (FDA) authorized food manufacturers to state on food labels that soy protein can help reduce the risk of heart disease. Studies show that soy can improve the elasticity of blood vessels and lower systolic blood pressure. Eat at least 25 grams of soy protein daily to realize a significant cholesterol-lowering effect. The FDA has stipulated that to qualify for heart-health claims, a food must contain at least 6.25 grams of soy protein per serving.

Soy is a good source of healthy carbohydrate, fiber, omega-3 fatty acids and protein. Soy products that supply protein include soy milk, tofu, soy flour, soy protein isolate, soy protein concentrate, textured soy protein or tempeh, soy-based meat substitute, fresh green soybeans and soy nuts.

## Protective Phytochemicals

It turns out that our mothers were right when they said, "Eat your fruits and vegetables." Evidence is mounting that the phytochemicals supplied by fruits and vegetables provide a natural protection from cancer, degenerative diseases and environmental toxicity. For example, cruciferous vegetables—broccoli, cabbage and Brussels sprouts—are major sources of phytochemicals and reduce the risk of developing bladder and other cancers. Tomatoes, which contain a phytochemical called lycopene, provide protection from prostate and other cancers.

Now, let's discuss the importance of vitamins and antioxidants.

# Chapter 27

## *Supplements, Vitamins and Antioxidants*

> Many health food stores might better be called pill
> stores, given how little food they stock in relation to
> all the vitamins and supplements. Claims made for
> these products are extravagant. If they were all true, we
> could forget about proper diet, exercise, relaxation, and
> all other preventive strategies and just take pills.
> – *Natural Health, Natural Medicine*
> Andrew Weil, M.D.

Optimal nutrition is fundamental to repairing, rebuilding and
restoring the health of your cells. This is even more important when
you suffer from IBS, because healthier cells augment the healing
process. You will benefit from a good multivitamin supplement, but
taking multivitamins is no substitute for eating a balanced and
healthy diet. Healthy foods—especially fresh fruits and vegetables—
contain phytochemicals and trace elements that are not available
in most multivitamins. Additionally, there are many healing substances in fruits, vegetables, nuts and grains that have not even been
isolated yet, and which are certainly missing from multivitamin
supplements.

## Multivitamins

Many people today, especially fast food lovers, do not get the nutrients
and trace elements they need. Many foods are stripped of their nutritional
value by microwaving, freezing, overcooking or frying. Sweets and junk

food fill you up with "empty calories" that have no nutritive value. For this reason, we recommend a good multivitamin supplement for most patients.

Most brands of multivitamins are perfectly safe. Many companies claim that natural vitamins are better than synthetic vitamins and charge more money for "natural" ingredients; however, no evidence shows that natural vitamins are superior to synthetic vitamins. Still, significant differences exist from brand to brand, particularly in how they are absorbed and in the amount of different vitamins, antioxidants and trace minerals they contain.

## Antioxidants and Free Radicals

Free radicals are toxic byproducts of oxygen metabolism that can cause significant damage to living cells and tissues in a process called "oxidative stress." The vitamins and minerals the body uses to counteract oxidative stress are called antioxidants.

Though free radicals are a normal byproduct of oxygen metabolism, certain environmental and behavioral risks dramatically increase the number of free radicals in the body, which in turn dramatically increases the oxidative stress on the body. Cigarette smoking is the most potent free radical generator in the body. Even one or two puffs sends the amount of oxidative stress on your body soaring. Environmental pollution, fried foods and charcoal broiled meats also increase oxidative stress. The resulting increase in free radicals can disrupt cell membranes, increase the risk of many forms of cancer and damage the interior lining of your blood vessels, leading to a higher risk of heart disease and stroke.

You can see how antioxidants work to counteract free radicals when you cut open an apple. Within minutes, the apple starts to turn brown due to the oxidative stress of free oxygen radicals in the air attacking the cells of the apple. If you take that same apple, slice it again and squirt lemon juice on it, the antioxidants in the lemon juice slow the oxidative process and keep the apple from turning brown.

The main antioxidants are vitamin A, beta-carotene (a water-soluble precursor to vitamin A), vitamin E, ascorbic acid (vitamin C) and the trace mineral selenium. These antioxidant vitamins can block the harmful effects of free radicals before cellular damage occurs. Population studies and clinical trials show lower rates of cancer and heart disease in populations eating foods high in antioxidant vitamins.

Expert opinion remains divided about whether taking antioxidant vitamins in dosages higher than the recommended daily allowance (RDA) confers additional benefits. We recommend the moderate approach given in Table 27.1.

---

Table 27.1

## Recommendations for Vitamins and Antioxidants

- Eat fruits and vegetables rich in antioxidant vitamins (sweet potatoes, spinach, carrots, broccoli, cantaloupe and citrus fruits).
- Take a good multivitamin that includes safe and effective amounts of the antioxidant vitamins and trace minerals.
- Don't take megadoses of vitamins unless you are under the care of a physician and registered dietician.
- If you decide to take antioxidants each day, then we recommend:
  - Vitamin C, 250 mg
  - Vitamin E, 400 to 800 IU of a natural form (d-alpha-tocopherol)
  - Selenium, 200 mcg of a yeast-bound type
  - Mixed carotenoids, 25,000 IU
  - B-complex vitamins that provide at least 400 mcg of folic acid
  - Calcium, 1,200 to 1,500 mg as calcium carbonate for those who are under 65 years of age or calcium citrate for those who are over 65 years of age.

---

Learn more about vitamins.

In the next chapter, you will learn about weight.

# Chapter 28
## *Weight*

**By any standard, it's alarming (referring to obesity).**
– Arthur Frank, M.D.
Medical Director, George Washington
University Obesity Management Program

> For the first time, more Americans are overweight than are at a
> healthy weight. Fifty-five percent of the adult population of the U.S.
> is considered to be overweight or obese. Obesity is the second lead-
> ing cause of preventable death in the United States. Three hundred
> thousand people die from obesity-related diseases every year. Obe-
> sity contributes to your allostatic load, so achieving and maintaining
> a healthy weight are important for your healing.

## Body Mass Index (BMI)

The National Institutes of Health has announced a new definition of
overweight and obesity based upon a calculation called the body mass
index or BMI. It relates body weight and height and is closely linked to
a person's body fat. You can determine your BMI with the following
formula.

Step 1.  Multiply your weight in pounds by 704.5.
Step 2.  Multiply your height in inches by your height in inches
(this is the square of your height).
Step 3.  Divide the answer in Step 1 by the answer in Step 2 to
calculate your BMI.

A BMI over 25 is considered overweight. Obesity is defined as a BMI of 31.1 or higher for males and 32.3 or higher for females.

Try our BMI calculator.

## Why Worry About Weight?

It is estimated that the average person gains at least one pound of fat and loses one-half pound of muscle each year beginning at age 20 unless he or she makes a lifestyle change. Excess body fat places you at high risk for heart disease, hypertension, stroke, diabetes, gallbladder disease, osteo-arthritis, sleep apnea, respiratory problems and certain cancers, especially of the breast and endometrium (uterus). Obesity is expensive, too. The National Institutes of Health estimates that obesity-related disease costs the nation approximately $100 billion each year.

## Losing Weight

Even a modest amount of weight loss is beneficial for most over-weight people, especially if other medical problems, such as hypertension, diabetes or high cholesterol, are present. Federal guidelines recommend that peo-ple maintain weight in a single healthy range instead of allowing weight to creep up over the years. Avoid crash weight loss by using a combination of exercise

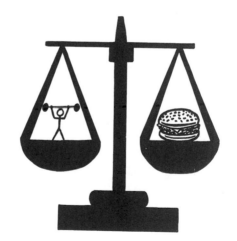

and healthy eating to achieve a slow and steady loss of weight (about ½ to 1 pound per week). Weight reduction of even 5% to 10% of body weight may improve many of the problems associated with being overweight, such as high blood pressure and diabetes.

Learn more about weight loss.

If you want online motivational help with your weight loss goals, visit Dr. Neimark's on-line self-help program called "You Can Do It!" at www.mindbodymed.com.

# Reward Your Efforts!

Self-care, wellness and relief from your IBS symptoms depend upon an effective weight management program. This requires that you make a commitment to a healthy diet and an exercise plan. Understanding the MindBodySpirit Connection is the key to successful weight management. Every single meal that you choose wisely and every day that you exercise well should be a cause for celebration. We all have ups, downs and diversions from our path toward greater health. Part of being successful at achieving any new goal is to fully celebrate the victories. We all tend to focus on what we don't have, the clothes we don't yet fit into and what we wish we looked like. Change your focus to an appreciation of the positive steps you are taking toward your goal. Reward your efforts by doing something you really enjoy (other than eating!) like buying a new CD, taking a warm bath or whirlpool or getting a massage. Celebrate your new body as it changes into the body you want it to become.

In the next two chapters, we'll discuss exercise.

# Chapter 29

## *Exercise*

Endurance exercise by itself can be a great stress reducer
and source of relaxation. But it has also been my experience
that a physical program works best when it's accompanied
by a tranquil mind and spirit.
— *It's Better to Believe*
Kenneth Cooper, M.D.
"Father of Aerobics"

For most people, exercise is an essential element of an effective plan
for self-care and wellness. IBS sufferers have even more to gain from
exercise because it can greatly relieve their symptoms. Weight control
based upon diet alone—without exercise—is uniformly unsuccess-
ful. However, exercise is beneficial in both losing and maintaining
weight, in converting fat to muscle and in increasing your metabolic
rate. Exercise is one of the best methods that you can use to reduce
your allostatic load.

Recent statistics from the National Institutes of Health (NIH) indicate
that 58% of American adults get little if any exercise and that more than
50 million American adults are completely sedentary. Former U.S. Surgeon General C. Everett Koop, M.D., has said that between 200,000
and 300,000 people die each year from the effects of a sedentary lifestyle. American sedentary behavior is a public health problem that results in aging complicated by obesity, diabetes, heart disease, infirmity
and frailty.

## Exercise Prescription

Exercise is an essential element of a plan for self-care and wellness and can be beneficial in managing IBS and other functional gut syndromes. Exercise will reduce your allostatic load. Here are some guidelines for including exercise in your life.

- The Centers for Disease Control and Prevention along with the American College of Sports Medicine recommend that all Americans accumulate 30 minutes or more of moderate-level physical activity on most and preferably all days of the week.
- Intermittent activity also confers substantial benefits. The 30 minutes of activity can be accumulated in short bouts of activity: walking up stairs instead of taking the elevator, walking instead of driving short distances or parking your car at the far end of the parking lot so you can walk further to get to the store.
- People who currently meet the recommended minimal standards of an accumulated duration of at least 30 minutes per day of moderate-intensity physical activity may derive additional health benefits by becoming more physically active or including more vigorous activity.

## Exercise and IBS: A Unique Challenge

The longest step in the journey is the first, so you—like most people—may be having difficulty motivating yourself to begin a life-long exercise program. It's even more difficult with your IBS. In the beginning, some forms of exercise may upset your stomach a bit, and that discomfort can be discouraging. But with time, exercise will reduce your IBS symptoms.

A gradual and incremental exercise program utilizing low impact aerobic activities like fast walking, biking, swimming or water aerobics is most likely to be successful. The type and intensity of the program may need to be individualized, and physical therapists or exercise specialists can provide helpful instruction (Chapter 40). You have much to gain (and weight to lose!) from starting an exercise program, if you will only take the first step.

| Important: Get a Medical Examination |
| --- |
| If you are a man over the age of 45 or a woman over age 55 and/or if you have heart disease or two or more cardiac risk factors, such as high blood pressure or cigarette smoking, you should consult with a physician before starting a program more vigorous than walking. |

# Aerobic Exercise and Resistance Training

Two types of exercise—aerobic and resistance—provide different and complementary benefits. Aerobic exercise (also called "cardio" or endurance exercise) will be discussed in this chapter. Resistance training (also called "weights" or strength training) will be discussed in the next chapter. Both types of exercise are important in a balanced exercise program, but we recommend that people with IBS and other functional GI disorders develop aerobic fitness first, over the course of 3 to 6 months, before beginning resistance training.

# Aerobic (Endurance or Cardio) Exercise

The term *aerobics* was introduced in 1968 by Kenneth Cooper, M.D. The book, called *Aerobics,* became an instant best seller and sparked the popularity of endurance exercise, leading to the commercial success of celebrities like Jane Fonda and Richard Simmons. Dr. Cooper defines aerobics as large-muscle endurance exercise that increases pulse and breathing rates for a prolonged period of time.

Just 30 minutes of walking each day has been shown to substantially reduce the risk of disease and relieve IBS symptoms. The benefits of walking are cumulative—three 10-minute walks are equivalent to one 30-minute walk. (This is true for exercise benefit, but not for weight loss benefit. To lose weight effectively, it is best that the entire exercise period occur at the same time.) Of all endurance exercises, walking is the most efficient way to burn fat. It is a weight-bearing activity that exercises the large muscle groups and requires the most calories. Walkers should move fast enough to notice their breathing, but slow enough to be able to carry on a conversation. On average, one hour of brisk walking burns 300 to 450 calories.

# Special Instructions for Getting Started

It can be difficult for IBS sufferers to start and maintain an exercise program; symptoms of pain and fatigue may seem to worsen when exercise is initiated. However, the ultimate value of an exercise program is substantial. Here are some special instructions for IBS sufferers.

- **Chart your progress.**  Record your progress in writing. You will be amazed at how helpful this step is in motivating you to continue.
- **Start slowly.**  If you are just beginning your program, you should walk, swim or cycle for no more than 5 minutes at a time. Do this at least 3 times a day if you can. Your goal will be to exercise on most days for at least 30 minutes.
- **Build gradually.**  Increase the length of your exercise sessions by about 10 percent each week. For example, if you are walking for 10 minutes a day for a week, increase to 11 minutes a day for the next week.
- **Challenge yourself without becoming discouraged.**  Remember that you are trying to get your heart to pump harder than it does at rest and eventually to break a light sweat. You may be somewhat out of breath, but you should be able to carry on a conversation while you exercise.
- **Weight loss is good if overweight.**  Carrying extra body weight is an unnecessary load that can fatigue your muscles and joints, so losing even 10% of your body weight can be beneficial. The best strategy for successful and permanent weight loss is exercise combined with healthy eating.
- **Develop endurance fitness before undertaking a resistance exercise program.**  You will be better prepared to begin building strength and muscle mass when your aerobic exercise program is well established.

You are now ready to learn about resistance exercise in the next chapter.

# Chapter 30

## *Resistance Exercise*

People don't exercise simply to improve their physical well-being or in an attempt to stay thin or stave off the effects of aging. They become dedicated to exercise because they find it helps them feel good emotionally and physically.
*– Mind Body Medicine*
Michael H. Sacks, M.D.

---

After developing aerobic fitness, we recommend that you move on to building muscle and strength. Research shows that you can accomplish the strength and muscular dimension of your self-care and wellness program in as little as 20 to 30 minutes, two to three times a week. Strength can be doubled, fat replaced with muscle—and most importantly for those with IBS—symptoms can be relieved through reduction of allostatic load.

---

## Creeping Obesity and Muscle Loss

Without engaging in resistance training, most adults lose muscle and gain fat as they age. Between the ages of 20 and 50, the average person loses ½ pound of muscle per year and replaces it with up to 1½ pounds of fat (Figures 30.1 and 30.2). So she or he loses 15 pounds of muscle and adds as much as 45 pounds of fat. This creeping obesity is often disguised by the shrinking muscle mass. Instead of a weight gain of 45 pounds, the loss of 15 pounds of muscle results in only 30 pounds of weight gain. However, many people gain more fat weight than that gained by the average person. Without resistance exercise training, if you never gain a pound of

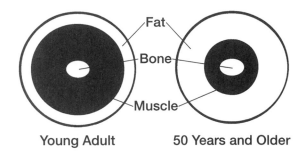

**Fat and Muscle Changes without Exercise**

**Figure 30.1**

weight between high school graduation and your 50th birthday, 15 pounds of your lost muscle will have been replaced by 15 pounds of fat. None of this is healthy.

## The Benefit of Muscle

Building muscle is important, especially if you want to lose weight. Adding muscle increases your body metabolism. Muscles burn most of the calories we eat. In fact, each pound of muscle you add to your body burns an extra 50 calories per day—that's 350 calories a week.

You build muscle through resistance training. Scientific studies confirm that resistance training—started at *any* age—counteracts age-related loss of muscle mass, improves strength and converts fat to muscle. Resistance training improves your ability to perform the activities of life and reduces your injury potential. Resistance training reduces your allostatic load.

## What Is Resistance Training?

You can use either free weights or machines as long as your large muscle groups are worked beyond their usual capacity. The American College of Sports Medicine recommends resistance training two to three times a week and flexibility workouts (discussed below) two to three times a week.

## Aging without Exercise: Fatter, Less Muscular

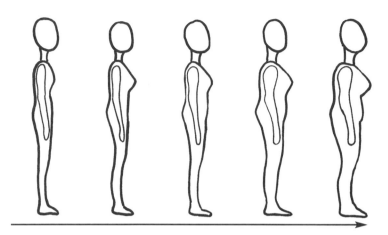

**Figure 30.2**

To build and maintain muscle, resistance training must be intense. Arthur Jones, the founder of Nautilus exercise machines, said, "The human body is exercised best, not by the volume of work but rather by the energy put momentarily into that work. Train harder, but briefer."

The resistance exercise program that we use and recommend is the one described by Ellington Darden, Ph.D., in his book written for men, *Living Longer Stronger,* and for women, *Body Defining.* His website is <u>www. classicx.com</u>. Dr. Darden's practical resistance-training program works all of the major muscle groups on the same day. You complete the entire workout in 30 minutes or less, two to three times a week. You do one set of each recommended exercise very slowly to the point at which the resistance (weight) can no longer be moved and another repetition is impossible. Another term that is used to describe this slow movement of the resistance to momentary muscular failure is "High Intensity Training."

# Stretching Workouts

It's a good idea to stretch before you exercise. Do light stretching as part of your warm-up, but wait until after your warm-up or for your cool-down

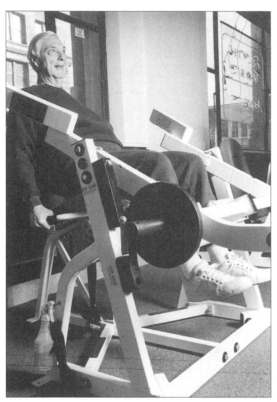
**Resistance Training Should Be Preceded by Stretching**

period to do more aggressive stretching. Research shows that holding a stretch for at least 30 seconds provides the most lasting benefits.

Stretching is a wonderful time to contemplate the health benefits you will enjoy from exercise. Visualize and imagine the level of physical, mental and spiritual vitality you will obtain as you work toward your health goals. Stretch your full mind, body and spirit in pursuit of your goals.

## A Final Word

Expect success. If you fear that the temporary discomfort of exercise will worsen your IBS, that's what is likely to happen. You need to overcome your fears in order to heal. If you are having a really bad bout of IBS, we recommend that you suspend your exercise program for a few days or exercise at 50% of your usual pace. Expect your pain to diminish and your confidence to build.

Be patient and progress gradually. If exercise causes discomfort, realize that the discomfort of exercise will not harm you. If you have pain, think of it as the labor pains of "giving birth" to a new and healthier you.

Learn more about <u>exercise</u>.

In the next chapter, we'll discuss the effects of alcohol, nicotine and caffeine.

# Chapter 31
## *Caffeine, Alcohol and Nicotine*

A custom loathsome to the eye, hateful to the nose,
harmful to the brain, dangerous to the lungs, and in
the black, stinking fume thereof, nearest resembling the
horrible Stygian smoke of the pit that is bottomless.
— *A Counterblast to Tobacco* (1604)
King James I

Caffeine, alcohol and nicotine interfere with sleep, which can contribute to the vicious cycle that perpetuates the symptoms of IBS. In addition, caffeine is a stimulant which can intensify anxiety and the pain and diarrhea of IBS. Smoking and/or excessive use of alcohol increase your allostatic load.

## Caffeine

Caffeine is a strong stimulant found in coffee, tea, chocolate, soft drinks and many over-the-counter medications and prescription drugs. It affects the brain, heart and GI system. Caffeine enhances the pain-relieving effects of aspirin or acetaminophen and for this reason it is added to some prescription headache medications. When combined with caffeine, the same amount of relief from pain is obtained using 40% less of the analgesic drug.

Caffeine can trigger the symptoms of IBS—especially abdominal cramping and diarrhea—as well as aggravate heartburn and dyspepsia. It does so by stimulating the gut directly; by stimulating the brain and heart, which contributes to anxiety; and by interfering with sleep. Many people do not realize that caffeine can cause or contribute to IBS, fibromyalgia, headache, jittery feelings, sleep disturbance, fatigue, malaise, irregular heart beat, panic and anxiety attacks.

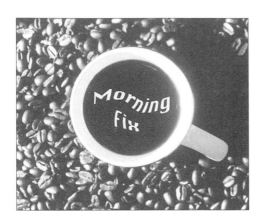

Table 31.1 lists the amount of caffeine in various foods. Serious side effects from caffeine can occur with as little as 250 mg per day, but many people with IBS or anxiety are susceptible to much lower levels, like the amount found in even one cup of coffee.

## Withdrawing from caffeine

The regular use of caffeine can lead to rebound or withdrawal headaches. To avoid withdrawal symptoms, reduce the amount of caffeine gradually. Begin with a 5-ounce reduction of coffee or cola every five to seven days until low doses are reached (100 to 120 mg per day). This dose can be maintained or discontinued altogether. Gradual withdrawal from caffeine can take up to several months.

Table 31.1

### Amounts of Caffeine for Various Sources

| Caffeine Sources | Milligrams of Caffeine |
| --- | --- |
| Brewed coffee (1 cup) | 100–150 |
| Instant coffee (1 cup) | 85–100 |
| Decaffeinated coffee (1 cup) | 2–4 |
| Tea (1 cup) | 30–40 |
| Cocoa (1 cup) | 40–55 |
| Cola (8 ounces) | 40–60 |
| Chocolate bar | 25 |

# Alcohol

Alcohol (especially beer) irritates the gut and causes diarrhea. Alcohol may also trigger IBS symptoms. It is worthwhile to try a period of abstinence from drinking to see if alcohol is one of your gut triggers/stressors. Alcohol can also interfere with sleep, disturbing your body's restorative capacity and thereby aggravating your IBS symptoms. Furthermore, excessive alcohol intake can damage the stomach and intestinal lining, causing ulcerations, gastritis and intestinal bleeding. 💻Learn more about <u>alcohol</u>.

# Nicotine and Tobacco

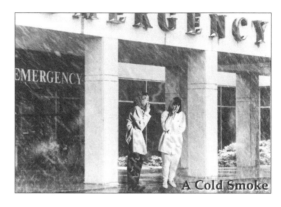

A Cold Smoke

All cigarette packs carry this Surgeon General's warning: "Quitting smoking now greatly reduces serious risks to your health." No health-related behavior is more self-destructive and adds more to allostatic load than smoking. Smoking is responsible for several hundred thousand deaths in the United States every year and is linked to several types of cancer, especially lung cancer. It causes and aggravates emphysema, chronic bronchitis and asthma and is associated with an increased risk of stroke, heart attack and impaired circulation. Smoking is inconsistent with a plan for self-care and wellness, and, because it can act as a gut trigger, may aggravate your IBS. The air swallowed during smoking can contribute to intestinal gas and cause heartburn, dyspepsia and indigestion. 💻Learn more about <u>smoking cessation</u>.

Now let's move on to the next step, where you will learn how to better care for your mind and spirit.

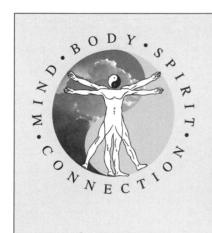

Addictive substances, such as caffeine, alcohol and nicotine, show the power of the MindBodySpirit Connection—for good and ill. You may begin to use a substance to satisfy emotional needs, but then find that you have become physically addicted and spiritually depleted. Mind, body and spirit are like a three-legged stool, especially when dealing with addiction. All three legs are necessary for stability and strength.

221

# STEP 6

## CARING FOR YOUR
## MIND AND SPIRIT

# Write From Your Heart

## TURNING POINTS

A JOURNAL OF NEW DIRECTIONS, WITH ILLUSTRATIONS AND QUOTES

### Health
### Healing
### Meaning

# Chapter 32

## *Self-Tests for Personal Problems*

**Distress and pain are friends to growth.**

– Augustus Napier

Now that you understand that personal problems, harmful stress, emotional hurts or painful memories may be contributing to your IBS, you realize that addressing these problems is vital to your recovery and healing. Healing always requires acknowledging "where you are"—mentally, emotionally, physically and spiritually—so that you may one day arrive at where you want to be.

The following tests are available on our website to help you determine if you have any of the five following problems that may interfere with your healing from IBS.

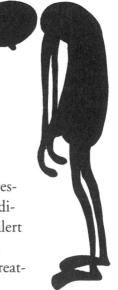

1. Alcohol abuse and alcoholism
2. Depression
3. Anxiety and Panic
4. Somatoform Disorder
5. Eating Disorder (Anorexia/Bulimia)

These screenings only indicate that a problem may be present. Your doctor needs to confirm any diagnosis with additional questioning and evaluation. Still, these tests may alert you to the possible presence of a problem and aid you in becoming a responsible partner in your own diagnosis, treatment and recovery. Learn more about <u>self-tests</u>.

Write your pain away in the next chapter.

# Chapter 33
## *Keeping a Journal*

Memory . . . is the diary that we all carry about with us.
— *The Importance of Being Earnest*
Oscar Wilde

Confessional writing has been recommended for healing since the Renaissance. New research scientifically confirms that writing about emotionally traumatic experiences is beneficial to your health and can reduce your allostatic load.

## Emotion, Thoughts and Stress

You have learned about the biological, psychological, social and spiritual aspects of illness. You have also seen how the effects of the accumulated bad stress response of allostatic load—whether you are consciously aware of it or not—can lead to an enhanced sensitivity of the gut and body to pain, resulting in unpleasant symptoms such as those experienced with IBS. By contrast, social support, love, connection with others and spirituality have a positive and buffering effect upon the bad stress response. In this chapter, we'll discuss another activity that can help you cope—journaling.

## Journaling

Journaling is the act of expressing your deepest thoughts and feelings by putting words to your inner life and then putting these words on paper. Journaling is a mental, emotional and spiritual exercise that helps you build strong "emotional muscles" to deal with life's difficulties and uncertainties. In identifying your negative thoughts and beliefs and

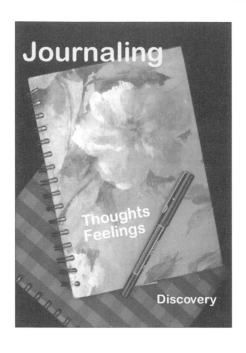

cultivating positive, healing ones in their place, journaling helps you discover your sense of purpose and meaning in life, as well as your relationship to a higher power.

Resilience to stress—even distress related to disease—is associated with how people manage their emotions. Realistic optimism can be helpful, but so is dealing directly with negative or hurtful feelings. In other words, suppressing painful feelings reduces your ability to experience any emotion, positive or negative.

Research has demonstrated that expressive writing about emotionally traumatic experiences (journaling) improves your health by releasing painful emotions and helping you change the meaning of your "story" about life or illness. A study published in 1999 in the *Journal of the American Medical Association* showed that writing about stressful life experiences improved symptoms of asthma and rheumatoid arthritis (1999;281:1304–1309). Learn more about <u>expressing feelings</u>.

## Writing Your Pain Away

An important use of journaling is processing your difficult emotions and stressful experiences before they lead to physical or emotional illness. Journaling helps you to recognize and manage your stress, alter the meaning of illness and overcome negative thought patterns. We offer three suggestions for expressive writing.

1. Write about your most stressful experiences and write from your heart. Don't keep a travelogue of events; write about your feelings and thoughts. A travelogue reads like this: "I woke up at 8 AM, went to walk the dog. I arrived late to work and my boss was angry with me." A journal entry looks like this: "I woke up feeling sad again. I don't know why. I am so upset by what happened at work

yesterday. I just don't want to face another day. It makes me so angry when they treat people unkindly. I can't stand it." Notice that a travelogue describes events, whereas a journal entry describes your feelings about events.

2. Ask yourself, "Was there something traumatic that happened in my life before the IBS began?" Or ask, "What happens emotionally in my life when my symptoms get worse?" Think carefully and be honest with yourself. Raising these questions and writing about them can help you to identify a relationship between your IBS and painful emotional events you may be unaware of.

3. Keep a daily journal for several weeks. This is an excellent way for you to get to know yourself better and enhance the connectedness of your mind, body and spirit. Keeping a journal can help you to take charge of your emotional and spiritual life and give you a sense of mastery and control over your thoughts, feelings, memories and life events. It may also help both you and your doctor find new ways for you to heal.

# Getting Started

The blank journal page on page 275 may be photocopied. Use one journal sheet every day for at least four weeks. Here are suggestions for constructing your journal.

## Symptoms

Rate the severity of your pain and fatigue from 0 to 10, with 0 being no symptoms and 10 being the worst possible symptoms. If you have other symptoms, list them and rate their severity. Rate your sleep as either good, fair, poor or none.

## Mind and life

Describe your thoughts, feelings, stresses, memories and what is happening in your life. This may lead you to recognize a correlation between life events and your symptoms.

## Analysis

Review your journal at least daily and more frequently if possible. In the space provided, evaluate your findings and observations. It is important to record not only your observations, but also your impressions about the relationship of your symptoms to your mental outlook and life events. Look for patterns and try to draw conclusions.

## Reprogramming statements

In addition to journaling, try changing your thought patterns into a more positive mode through reprogramming statements. Each of the following statements will help you to reprogram negative thoughts into positive ones. Put them in a place where you will see them often, and read them daily. Write a different one down each day until all seven are recorded, and memorize them if you wish. Make up statements that speak to you. Do this each week that you keep the journal. Here are some sample reprogramming statements.

1. My mind, body and spirit are one. I am healing one step at a time and that is good enough in this moment.
2. I cannot control the wind, but I can redirect my sails. I am reaching my goals for healing and peace of mind.
3. I am in control of my peace. Though my symptoms are disturbing, I will not let them rob me of my peace.
4. I did not cause my IBS, but I am gaining a sense of mastery over it.
5. I am courageously exploring all my stresses, feelings, memories and thoughts—so that I may heal my hurts and restore my health and peace of mind.
6. I am using my IBS to get to know myself, grow and become healthier than ever before.
7. I acknowledge my power to heal and accept responsibility for my health.

Learn more about journaling.

In the next chapter, you will learn other techniques for managing stress.

# Chapter 34

## *Stress Management and Relaxation Techniques*

> Breath is the link between the body and mind
> and between the conscious and unconscious mind.
> It is the master key to the control of emotions and
> to operations of the involuntary (autonomic)
> nervous system.
> — *8 Weeks to Optimum Health*
> Andrew Weil, M.D.

Scientific studies have confirmed that relaxation methods really do work and can help you manage your IBS. All stress management techniques aim to induce a positive parasympathetic state through the MindBodySpirit communication systems described in Step 2.

In 1996, a 12-member National Institutes of Health (NIH) panel representing the fields of family medicine, social medicine, psychiatry, psychology, public health, nursing and epidemiology, along with 23 other experts, concluded that a number of existing well-defined behavioral and relaxation interventions are effective in treating chronic pain and insomnia. The NIH panel found strong evidence for the use of relaxation techniques in reducing chronic pain in a variety of medical conditions (*JAMA,* 1996;276:313–318). We'll discuss some of these techniques in this chapter.

# The Breathing Technique

Andrew Weil, M.D.—a renowned authority on MindBody interactions—emphasizes that breathing can exert a strong influence on mind, body and mood. Directing attention to breathing moves you in the direction of relaxation. In his book, *Natural Health, Natural Medicine,* Dr. Weil writes, "The single most effective relaxation technique I know is conscious regulation of breath."

One simple breathing technique you can try involves breathing in deeply through your nose to a count of 8, holding your breath to a count of 8 and then exhaling through your mouth to a count of 8. Repeat this exercise 10 to 20 times or until you feel your body and mind relax. Other breathing ratios you can try are: In 8, Hold 8, Exhale 16; or In 8, Hold 16, Exhale 16.

# The Relaxation Response

The relaxation response was initially described by Herbert Benson, M.D., and his colleagues at Harvard Medical School in the early 1970s and most recently in his book *Timeless Healing: The Power and Biology of Belief.* Eliciting the relaxation response helps reverse the harmful effects of overstimulation of the body's automatic stress response (the fight-or-flight response) discussed in Step 2. While the body's fight-or-flight response is automatic and unconscious, the relaxation response must be intentionally and consciously elicited by simple mental techniques. It will take awhile before you feel the relaxation, but with practice the beneficial bodily changes are measurable and predictable. In some ways, practicing the elicitation of the relaxation response is like learning how to swim. You don't learn how to swim in a stormy ocean. Likewise, don't try to learn the relaxation response during very stressful times. We recommend learning to elicit the relaxation response under calm conditions. Later, it will help calm you under adverse conditions.

In reviewing the historical writings of ancient philosophies and religions, Dr. Benson found that throughout the ages, almost all religions and cultures had some form of meditative or prayerful ritual capable of eliciting the body's relaxation response. All of these varied techniques include two simple steps:

1. Focusing the mind on a repetitive word, sound, prayer, phrase or muscular activity, such as breathing.
2. Adopting a passive attitude toward the thoughts that go through your head. In other words, when intrusive thoughts come into your mind, you calmly disregard them and return your attention to the word or phrase you are repeating.

## Benefits to MindBodySpirit

Practicing the two simple steps above reliably and predictably elicits your body's relaxation response, which diminishes the harmful effects of excess allostatic load. Beneficial effects include:

- Immediate benefits—which occur as you focus upon a repetitive word, phrase, breath or action—include lowered blood pressure, heart rate, breathing rate and oxygen consumption (which means that your metabolic rate drops).
- Long-term benefits—which occur after practicing for at least a month—persist even when a person is not practicing the relaxation response, and appear to be due to an alteration of the body's response to epinephrine (the stress hormone made by the adrenal gland). The regular elicitation of the relaxation response can result in a reduction in anxiety/depression, functional MindBodySpirit symptoms and improvement in your ability to cope with stress.
- Spiritual benefits include a sense of increased spirituality. Harvard research has confirmed that people who elicited the relaxation response experienced the close presence of a higher power, force, energy or perception of God.

The relaxation response is not a technique, but rather a set of bodily responses that occur when a part of your brain is stimulated (the hypothalamus of the limbic system within the neuromatrix). When specific parts of your hypothalamus are electrically stimulated, all the positive physiologic benefits of the relaxation response occur. Since you can't implant an electrode in your brain, we recommend that you use Dr. Benson's simple technique to mentally stimulate these brain centers. When you practice the mental technique for 15 minutes, the physiologic changes that occur are measurable and predictable, whether you "feel" the technique is working, or not. Research shows that you will predictably derive the physiologic benefits of the relaxation response, whether you believe it works or not.

# Relaxation vs. Relaxation Response

Some people think that with a relaxation technique they will immediately feel relaxed. Many people who elicit the relaxation response do feel immediate relaxation, but for some it takes several months of practice before they actually feel relaxed. Remember, whether you "feel" it or not, invoking the relaxation response predictably lowers your blood pressure, decreases your oxygen consumption, relaxes your brain waves, lowers your respiratory rate and counteracts the harmful effects of the fight-or-flight response. According to Dr. Benson, eliciting the relaxation response should be like brushing your teeth; don't do it because it feels good, do it because you know it is good for you. Don't expect some mind-altering euphoria, just know that when you sit and practice the technique, the benefits to your body, mind and spirit predictably occur.

Being relaxed and eliciting the relaxation response are not the same unless being relaxed includes both a focus upon a repetitive stimulus and a passive attitude. The relaxation response is not obtained by reading a book, listening to quiet music, sleeping or "taking it easy." Though these activities may be relaxing to you, they do not bring about the beneficial physiologic changes of the relaxation response.

### Eliciting your body's relaxation response

Here is Dr. Benson's technique for eliciting your body's relaxation response. Don't be intimidated by all the steps. They all boil down to two basic things: (1) focus on a word or phrase that is meaningful or inspirational to you and (2) when your attention drifts or intruding thoughts enter your mind, disregard them and refocus on your word or phrase. It's really simple. Here is a more detailed step by step approach.

Step 1.   Pick a focus word or short phrase that is firmly rooted in your belief system.

Step 2.   Sit quietly in a comfortable position.

Step 3.   Close your eyes.

Step 4.   Relax your muscles.

Step 5.   Breathe slowly and naturally, and as you do, repeat your focus word or phrase silently to yourself as you exhale.

Step 6.   Assume a passive attitude. Don't worry about how well you're doing. When other thoughts come to mind, simply say to yourself, "Oh, well," and gently return to the repetition.

Step 7.   Continue for 10 to 20 minutes.

Step 8.   Do not stand immediately. Continue sitting quietly for a minute or so, allowing other thoughts to return. Then open your eyes and sit for another minute before rising.

Step 9.   Practice this technique once or twice daily.

Reprinted with the permission of Scribner, a Division of Simon & Schuster Inc., from TIME-LESS HEALING: THE POWER AND BIOLOGY OF BELIEF by Herbert Benson, M.D., with Marg Stark. Copyright © 1996 by Herbert Benson, M.D.

The relaxation response can also be evoked with your eyes open and in other body positions, like standing or lying down.

## Exercise and the relaxation response

The relaxation response can be elicited during repetitive exercise, such as walking, jogging or swimming by paying attention to the cadence of the repetitive movement in the exercise, like the sound of your feet hitting the pavement. With each repetitive movement, silently repeat in your mind the special word or phrase you have chosen. Unfocused exercise, like riding a bike while listening to a walkman or running on a treadmill while watching TV, will not invoke the relaxation response. You must pay attention to the rhythm of the exercise and consciously repeat the word or phrase silently in your mind while disregarding all intrusive thoughts by returning to your word or phrase when you catch yourself drifting. Many people who have trouble relaxing or sitting still will benefit from this more active method for eliciting the relaxation response. Remember that exercise is beneficial in stress management even without the application of the relaxation response because it metabolizes excess stress hormones from your body. But try exercising with the relaxation response for even more benefit.

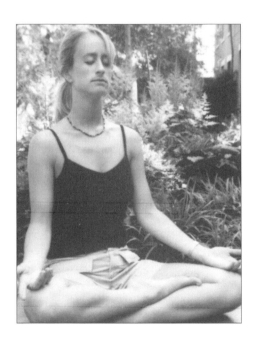

## Yoga

Yoga is a combination of exercise and mental relaxation. It is really a form of moving meditation and conscious breathing. Yoga is a superb, low impact form of stretching, exercise and breathing that yields phenomenal health benefits for your mind, body and spirit.

## Laughter

Josh Billings, a nineteenth century humorist, said, "There ain't much fun in medicine, but there's a heck of a lot of medicine in fun." There is strong scientific evidence that the opposite of the stress response is laughter and that the beneficial changes that occur in the body from laughter are real and measurable. Norman Cousins emphasized this in his book *Anatomy of an Illness*, in which he used humor and laughter to recover from a serious disease. He reported that ten minutes of solid belly laughter would provide him with two hours of pain-free sleep. The popular movie *Patch Adams* (1998) makes the same point. Duke University has prepared a list of humorous materials available to its patients.

Learn more about <u>stress management</u>.

In the next chapter, we'll discuss how cognitive-behavioral therapy can help you manage your IBS.

# Chapter 35
## *Cognitive Behavioral Therapy*

**If you don't control your mind, someone else will.**
– John Allston

**Ya gotta wanna.**
– Robert Sherer

Cognitive therapy is based on the work of Aaron T. Beck, M.D., a world authority on mood disorders. The word *cognitive* refers to how you think about things at any particular moment. Dr. Beck's thesis is simple: When you are depressed or anxious, you may be thinking in an irrational, self-defeating manner that limits your choices and your sense of hope. When you make an effort to retrain yourself and think differently about situations, you can reduce your physical and emotional symptoms and reduce your level of distress. This process is called a "mental tune-up."

## Principles of Cognitive Therapy

The first principle of cognitive therapy is that the majority of your moods are created by your thoughts, perceptions, attitudes and beliefs about a situation. They are not caused by the actual situation itself. That is, you feel the way you do in any given moment because of the thoughts you are thinking and the meaning you give those thoughts. Your thoughts—whether you are conscious of them or not—create your mood.

The second principle is that when you feel stressed-out, anxious or depressed, your thoughts are often irrational, negative or based on distorted perceptions. Cognitive behavioral therapy helps you identify your distorted thoughts and perceptions.

## Cognitive Journaling

Journaling about your feelings with the intent of identifying the irrational, negative or distorted thoughts and perceptions that accompany them is called cognitive journaling. Cognitive journaling helps you identify and revise your distorted perceptions and irrational thoughts. Follow these cognitive journaling steps and see if they help. This whole process can be considered one of keeping an "emotional accounting" of your life. This is as important as keeping your checkbook balanced! Maybe more important!

1. Every time you feel depressed, anxious or conflicted, write down your emotional response: depressed, angry, sad, afraid, frustrated, hopeless and so on.
2. Try to identify the thoughts that precede or accompany your emotional reaction.
3. Next, identify the irrational component, negative distortion or illogical part of the thought. (See "List of Cognitive Distortions.")
4. Now *breathe, reflect* and *choose* a rational response to the automatic negative thoughts. Write the rational response down.
5. Lastly, revisit the initial emotional or physical reaction you had and see if the intensity has decreased, increased or stayed the same.

### A Cognitive Journaling Example

1. Emotional Response: "I feel depressed today. My stomach is tied up in knots."
2. Corresponding Thought: "I will never get relief from my IBS. I am going to suffer forever."
3. Cognitive Distortion: You identify this illogical thought as a form of "All or Nothing" thinking (i.e., "I will always suffer.").
4. Breathe, reflect and choose a rational response: "Yes, I am having an exceptionally bad day today, but I have many good days with few or no symptoms. I know I can get through this."
5. With the realization that your symptoms are temporary, you revisit your feelings of depression. Now you don't feel as depressed and are able to focus on the good things in store for today.

# Cognitive Distortions

Here is a list of the most common cognitive (thought) distortions. Can you identify any of them in yourself?

1. All-or-Nothing Thinking
2. Overgeneralization
3. Mental Filter: Picking out a single negative detail and ignoring other aspects
4. Disqualifying the Positive
5. Jumping to Conclusions: Mind Reading or The Fortune Teller Error
6. Magnification ("catastrophizing") or Minimization
7. Emotional Reasoning: I feel it, therefore it must be true.
8. Should Statements
9. Labeling and Mislabeling: An extreme form of overgeneralization ("I'm a loser.")
10. Personalization: Claiming responsibility for negative events you didn't cause.

# Cognitive Behavioral Treatment

Managing chronic pain and functional symptoms requires an exploration of the relationship between your thoughts (mind/brain) and your symptoms (body). The source of thoughts and feelings is the mind/brain, which gives meaning to experience, including symptoms and pain. The mind acts as a filter or lens through which bodily messages of pain or discomfort pass. The filter or lens can either reduce or magnify the intensity of the message. Thus, the experience of pain and uncomfortable symptoms can be increased or decreased by the power of your mind. By changing your mind, you can change your brain chemistry and find relief from your symptoms (Figure 35.1 on the next page).

Cognitive-behavioral therapy gives you a set of practical tools that allow you to become more aware of self-defeating thoughts or beliefs that

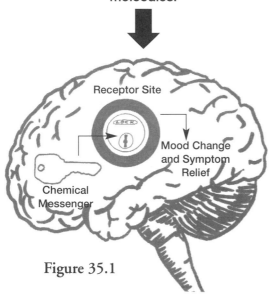

Thoughts, beliefs, memories, expectations, relaxation, exercise, diet, sleep and medication all create chemical messenger molecules.

Receptor Site

Mood Change and Symptom Relief

Chemical Messenger

**Figure 35.1**

may be contributing to your pain and discomfort. Many self-defeating thoughts are buried in your unconscious mind. Cognitive-behavioral therapy gives you the tools to bring these unconscious thoughts into conscious awareness, where you can correct your thought distortions and self-defeating behaviors and bring about positive and lasting change.

# Getting Cognitive Behavioral Treatment

Virtually everyone can benefit from cognitive behavioral therapy. You can learn these techniques either by working with a health-care professional (psychologist, psychiatrist, MFCC or social worker) or by using materials such as Dr. Margaret Caudill's book, *Managing Pain Before It Manages You,* or *Life Strategies: Doing What Works; Doing What Matters,* by Phillip C. McGraw, Ph.D. Learn more about <u>cognitive behavioral therapy</u>.

Even though you can resolve some issues on your own, it may be advisable to have a professional therapist or mental health provider help you. We all have blind spots especially when dealing with recurrent situations or painful memories. For this reason, it is always best to "reality check" your own self-help insights with an objective and concerned professional.

The next chapter will show you how to change your negative attitudes and beliefs.

# Chapter 36
## Changing Attitudes and Beliefs

**The important thing is this: To be able at any moment
to sacrifice what we are for what we could become.**
– Charles du Bois

You can learn effective ways to change your attitudes and beliefs by
learning to challenge the negative thoughts and irrational beliefs you
hold about yourself when bad things happen to you. With the
ABCDE technique that you will learn in this chapter, you can
achieve a level of healthy optimism and hopefulness that will help
you live a life of greater joy and wellness, minimizing the harmful
effects of trigger/stressor situations that you must sometimes face
because of your IBS.

One of the most respected researchers in
healthy attitudes is Martin Seligman, Ph.D.,
psychologist and author of *Learned Optimism.*
Dr. Seligman studied a condition called
"learned helplessness." He found that when
dogs were given unavoidable, inescapable
shocks, they seemed to give up even trying to
escape future shocks. That is, when they were
given a chance to escape the shocks by jumping over a low barrier, they acted helpless and
continued to accept the shocks. It was as if the
dogs actually learned to be helpless. If the animals had the chance to escape from the start,
they did not give up when they received future

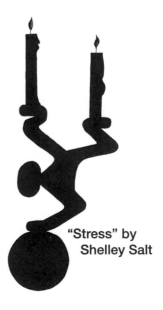

"Stress" by
Shelley Salt

shocks; they did not become helpless. Instead, they figured out a way to escape the shocks.

Using his observations on learned helplessness, Dr. Seligman created a scale to measure this characteristic in humans. He then devised an experiment where he rated 172 undergraduates for learned helplessness. Using this scale, he was able to accurately predict which students would become sick in the subsequent six months. In another study of 13 patients with malignant melanoma, he showed that the absence of learned helplessness was a better predictor of survival than the level of NKCA (Natural Killer Cell Activity), an important immune predictor in the bloodstream.

Dr. Seligman's work is a powerful testimonial to the need to guard against learned helplessness and find ways to release yourself from the unavoidable shocks of life. Remember that feeling helpless is a learned phenomenon and anything that is learned can be unlearned.

# The Three P's

You can learn how to overcome your learned helplessness by taking steps to reduce your stress response, taking control of your environment and developing positive attitudes. Your ability to overcome learned helplessness does not simply rely on positive thinking. It relies on your ability to challenge the negative attitudes and pessimistic beliefs you hold about yourself when bad things happen to you. In his research, Dr. Seligman discovered three conditions that characterize learned helplessness, called the Three P's:

1. We tend to take things *personally* and blame ourselves when bad things happen to us.
2. We tend to think that because one bad thing happened in one area of our life, that this negativity will become *pervasive* and affect all areas of our life.
3. We tend to believe that this one bad thing that happened to us means that we are forever flawed in this area and doomed to *permanent* failure.

In order to overcome learned helplessness, you must challenge the Three P's by: (1) learning not to take things so *personally* and attempting to find other explanations for the bad things that happen; (2) learning to see the limited nature of the adversity, realizing that it is not *pervasive,* but applies only to one small area of your life; and (3) attacking the negative assumption that your problem is *permanent* by allowing yourself to see the temporary nature of the adversity.

---

### An Example of the ABCDE Process

Johnny is having a bad day at work because his IBS is acting up. He feels uncomfortable and has less patience than usual. His short fuse causes him to yell at one of his difficult and argumentative customers in public. Johnny has always been a good worker in the past but after his outburst, he goes into a panic and is sure he will lose his job. He apologizes to the customer, but nevertheless, Johnny cannot let go of his anxiety about the situation. It continues to haunt him and deplete his energy and self-esteem.

Johnny can address his anxiety and overcome his learned helplessness by writing out the ABCDEs of the situation.

A. *Adversity:* Johnny yells at a customer.
B. *Beliefs:* "I am out of my mind." "I don't know how to get along with people."
C. *Consequences:* (of his negative beliefs) "I'll never be able to hold a job. I'm a loser. I'm sure I'll be fired."
D. *Dispute:* "I only lost it this one time. It's never happened before. I don't feel good today—my IBS is acting up and this is a really difficult customer. I can learn more about dealing with difficult customers so this doesn't happen again. I am generally a respectful and 'in-control' person. I can learn new ways to minimize my symptoms of IBS or do a deep breathing exercise to relax."
E. *Energize:* Johnny feels better having attacked his irrationally negative beliefs about the situation and he stops taking the problem so *personally,* realizing it is a temporary setback (not *permanent*) and that it is limited to this one incident and is not *pervasive.*

# Challenging Negative Beliefs

You can change your negative thinking to positive thinking with the ABCDE method. First, when *Adversity* strikes, examine the *Beliefs* you hold about the situation. Then look at the *Consequences* of your beliefs. When you see the negative consequences of your pessimistic attitudes and helpless beliefs, *Dispute* them by rationally attacking your negative beliefs. You do this by challenging the Three P's. Then, allow yourself to feel *Energized* by your new positive beliefs and celebrate your success! The ABCDE technique is a variant of the cognitive journaling method presented in the previous chapter.

Good luck with your ABCDEs! Now let's take a look in the next chapter at how you can cultivate a deeper sense of spirituality to help you heal your IBS symptoms.

# Chapter 37
## *Spirituality*

The greatest mistake in the treatment of disease is
that there are physicians for the body and physicians
for the soul, although the two cannot be separated.

– Plato

In its simplest form, MindBodySpirit medicine teaches that you are
a whole person, not just some "body" that is ill or diseased. The
MindBodySpirit connection teaches that everyone is composed of
two basic elements: a *body* (with physical limitations) and a *soul*
(with limitless possibilities). The function of your *mind* is to balance
the needs of your body with the needs of your soul.

## The Body/Soul Connection

In order to achieve optimal health, you must nurture and nourish both
your body and your soul. You nourish your body by listening to its needs
and honoring it through proper rest, nutrition and exercise. You nourish
your soul by transcending your own personal needs in order to reach out
and help others in need. When you begin to listen to your body, it teaches
you what you need. When you begin to listen to your soul, it teaches you
how you are needed.

MindBodySpirit medicine teaches that to create a meaningful life you
must unite your body and soul in a way that allows you to use your unique
talents and special gifts to make the world a kinder, more loving and more
beautiful place in which to live. This is the essence of MindBodySpirit medicine: that by channeling the physical energy of your body into noble and
transcendent pursuits of the soul, you create a meaningful life, one filled
with the sense of purpose, vitality and aliveness that characterize true health.

# The Wings of Your Soul: A Story*

A great Master once asked his gifted students to pursue not only their academic studies but also their spiritual studies—so that they would learn the importance of improving their character and practicing good deeds. One student anxiously replied to his Master that his schedule was already too full and there was no possible way he could help. Then, he looked at his Master and began to feel embarrassed, realizing that the Master's schedule was far busier than his own. Appreciating his dilemma, he asked the Master, "How do you do it Master? How do you have the strength and stamina to work as hard as you do?" The Master replied, "Every person has both a body and a soul. It is like a bird and its wings. Imagine—if a bird were unaware that its wings enabled it to fly, they would only add an extra burden of weight. But once it flaps its wings, it lifts itself skyward. We all have wings—our soul—that can lift us as high as we need go. All we have to do is learn to use them."

*The Master in this story is Rabbi Menachem Mendel Schneerson and this story is adapted from the book *Toward a Meaningful Life: The Wisdom of the Rebbe Menachem Mendel Schneerson.*

# Spiritual Practice

In order to spiritually fly, you must first flap your wings. This usually involves some form of spiritual practice or ritual that puts you in touch with soulfulness. The only way to develop your soul, nurture a relationship with a higher power and find a sense of purpose or meaning in life is to engage in spiritual exercise on a regular basis. Here are some forms:

- *Prayer:* Spend 10 to 15 minutes every day praying. Pray for the health and welfare of your loved ones. Pray for the strength to meet life's challenges. Pray for your physical, mental, emotional and spiritual needs.
- *Study holy books:* Spend 15 minutes a day reading scriptural passages from holy books like the Torah, the Bible, the Koran, the Bhagavad Gita and the like.

- *Practice gratitude:* Keep a gratitude journal. Remember that in the midst of your pain and trials there is much to be grateful for. Take five minutes at the end of the day to focus the camera of your mind on all the things you have to be grateful for.

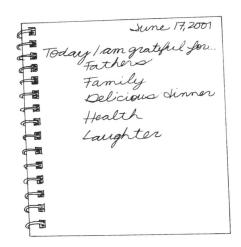

- *Attend church or synagogue:* Studies show that those who are religiously in-volved have less depression, less anxiety, less fear, greater marital stability, de-creased drug and alcohol abuse and a greater sense of purpose, well-being, hope and optimism in life.

- *Volunteer your time:* Remember that the essence of spirituality lies in your ability to reach beyond your own self-centered ideas, con-cerns and desires and connect with something outside yourself. Helping those in need is a wonderful way to flap the wings of your soul and lift yourself skyward, giving you a greater sense of belong-ing to the world.

- *Find and nurture your relationship with God or a higher power:* You don't have to fully comprehend the idea of God or a higher power to begin to develop a relationship with one. As in your own personal relationships, you usually get to know and love people most through the process of having a relationship with them. If you want to realize the presence of a higher power in your life, then you must make the effort to include a higher power in your life. Spending time with one another is the only way any relationship grows strong. Having a healthy relationship with God or with your higher power is no different. Be willing to speak to your higher power when you are upset or angry, and even fight with your higher power when nec-essary, but always with the goal of creating greater love and under-standing in the relationship.

- *Practice kindness:* Remember that part of everyone's higher purpose in life is practicing higher values—honoring the sacredness, worth and dignity of each individual. Make a conscious effort to practice kindness. When you act kindly and love others as yourself, you develop your soulfulness.

- *Create a life of meaning by finding your higher purpose:* The *New York Times* once printed an article on an elementary school teacher who had written a beautiful phrase on the chalkboard for her students to read. It said, "We're all gifted. Some of us just open up our packages sooner than others." You are gifted. You were given special qualities, talents and gifts that make you different and unique. In order to flap the wings of your soul, you must discover your unique gifts and use them in a meaningful way to help make the world a kinder, more loving and more beautiful place. Without this sense of contribution, this sense of purpose, you will never be able to live a truly meaningful and vitally healthy life. One of Neil's personal mentors, Richard A. Nyberg, Mdiv., MSW, says, "Do what you love that makes you more loving." This is the essence of finding a higher purpose.

- *Do good deeds:* Help others in need. Give them time. Give them money. Give them love. Share the many blessings you have been given. Take the extra moment to open the door for someone or lend a helping hand. Thinking virtuous thoughts is not enough—you must practice virtuous acts.

- *Read poetry and listen to inspirational music:* Nothing speaks to the soul like music and poetry. Music bypasses all your psychological defenses and speaks directly to your soul. The same is true of poetry. Soulful poetry penetrates the heart first, and only later does your head figure it out. Let the words of poets touch your heart and soul.

- *Practice honesty:* Practice honesty in all your dealings—with yourself and with others. Nothing lifts your wings skyward faster. Honesty is an essential quality of the soul. Be honest with yourself about what you feel and think. Be honest with others. Yes, it's risky, but there is no other way to truly heal. When you are dishonest with yourself or others, you hide parts of yourself that are essential for healing.

- *Spend time outdoors:* Reconnecting with the natural world elevates the soul by reminding us of cycles larger than ourselves—Earth's cycles. Plant a garden. Walk in a park. Go camping. Sit quietly and listen to the birds. Like the birds, your soul, too, can take wing.

These are just a few of the spiritual exercises that can help you flap the wings of your soul and lift yourself skyward in your journey of health and healing. Learn more about spirituality.

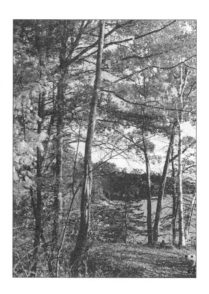

For inspirational messages on MindBodySpirit medicine or to sign up for Dr. Neimark's free newsletter, visit his website at: http://www. TheBodySoulConnection.com.

You have come a long way in your journey through this book, but if your symptoms persist, take the final step.

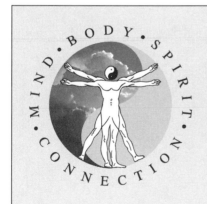

Spiritual needs are often put on the back burner. We don't take the time we need to rest and recharge. For this reason, we recommend that you literally make an appointment—with yourself—to stop and smell the roses. Take a walk. Look around you. Listen to the sounds in your neighborhood and smell the smells. Your mind, body and spirit will thank you!

# STEP 7

## TAKING ACTION IF SYMPTOMS PERSIST

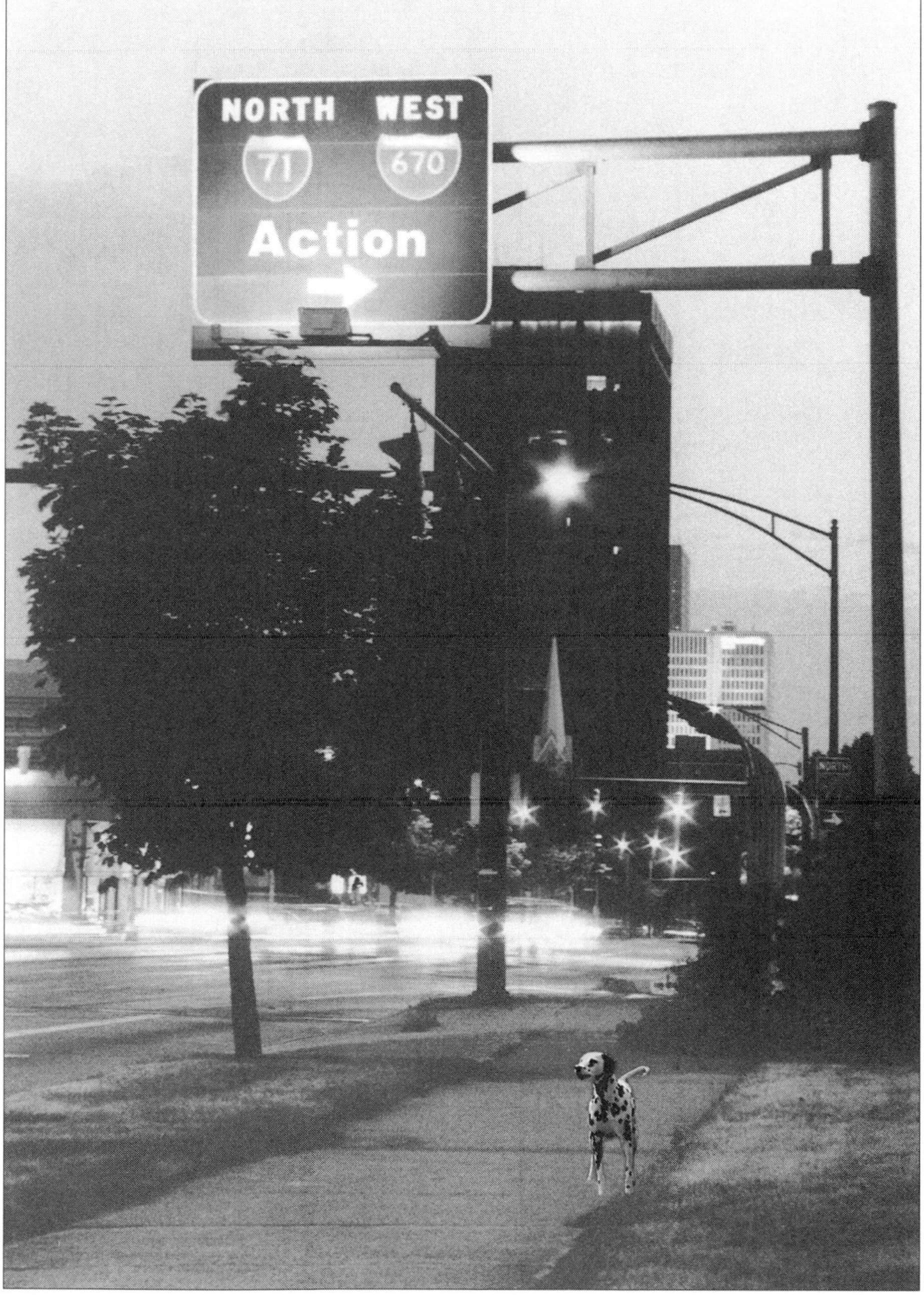
NORTH WEST
71 670
Action

# Chapter 38

## *Healing as a Process*

It is not simply mind over matter,
but it is clear that mind matters.
– David Spiegel, M.D.

The greatest revolution of our time is the
knowledge that human beings, by changing
the inner attitudes of their minds, can
transform the outer aspects of their lives.
– William James

> If a precious jewel accidentally fell into the mud, you would have to slowly chip away at the dirt, facet by facet, until you uncovered the precious and shining jewel hidden within. Healing is like chipping away at the attitudes, beliefs, memories, worries and stresses that obscure the precious core of who you are—the authentic you—the priceless jewel within that is deserving and ready to heal. Some parts of you are already shining through, while other parts lie waiting to be uncovered. Healing is the process of revealing your authentic self— the precious core of who you are—worthy and lovable.

## You Can't Read Your Way to Healing

It is critical that you really incorporate all that you have learned into an action plan for health and wellness. Reading about exercise will not make your body strong, and reading about the MindBodySpirit Connection will not make your IBS better. Stephen Levine, author of *Healing into Life and Death,* tells the story of a man who thought he could learn everything by reading. He read a book on astronomy and became an astronomer. He read a book on biology and became a biologist. He read a book on swimming and drowned. As this story illustrates, you can't read your way to healing. You must incorporate what you read by taking action and exerting the full force of your will and determination to heal.

# Honesty

Honesty is a vital element in any MindBodySpirit approach to healing. You must be completely honest with yourself regarding your feelings, your pain and your hurts. The honest expression of who you are is more important than pretending to be upbeat or positive. Margaret Kemeny, Ph.D., in *Healing and the Mind* (by Bill Moyers) found that the *honest expression* of emotion, whether it be negative (fear, anger, resentment and jealousy) or positive (happiness, peacefulness, joy and laughter) results in an increase in the number and activity of natural killer cells. "Positive thinking" will not keep you well, nor will "negative thinking" necessarily make you ill. Instead, be honest about what you feel and think, and express that honesty kindly and lovingly to yourself and others.

If you are not reaching the level of health and well-being you desire, ask yourself if you are being true to yourself. Do your behaviors grow from the roots of your being? Are you living your very own life, or are you trying to live the life everyone else wants you to live? You can't heal and develop your fullness of expression if you don't know who the real you is. You can't live your very own life if you are too busy living someone else's.

Learn more about <u>honesty and health</u>.

# Realistic Expectations

If your IBS symptoms are not improving as quickly as you had hoped, check your expectations. Are your expectations for healing and improvement realistic? Remember that the body always has some limitations and perfect health is unattainable. But you can expect to find a reasonable measure of peace, balance and serenity in a world filled with imperfection and endless uncertainty.

One definition of stress is the gap between expectations and reality. If your expectations are unrealistic—if you are trying to be or feel perfect all the time—you will always be unhappy and you will never reach the fullness of expression that is your birthright. Accept some of your limitations while continuing to seek new ways to heal and grow. This is the way to peace.

## Don't Do It Alone

Remember that no one can do it alone. We all need one another. If you are doing the best you can on your own—managing your stress, cultivating spirituality, exercising and eating well—and you are still not feeling well, then it is time to seek out others who can help you. We all need help from others to learn, grow and achieve important goals in life. At times, we all need others to nurture and care for us, especially when we have exceeded our ability to care for ourselves.

The next several chapters will introduce you to specialists, "centers of excellence" and resources for additional information and support that can offer you multidisciplinary and comprehensive help. To heal more deeply, you may want to consult a bodyworker to help you heal your body, a therapist to help you heal your mind and a spiritual mentor (minister/priest/pastor/rabbi/guru) to help you heal your soul.

But before you go on to learn more about these healers, consider some of the following suggestions to help you move to the next level of healing.

- Review Step 1 and think about the power of MindBodySpirit medicine and healing. Are you "using" your IBS symptoms to learn more about yourself and your stressors/triggers? Or, are you just taking on more and more allostatic load? Are you learning how to accept some of the limitations of your body while discovering the limitless possibilities of your soul? Have you incorporated spirituality into your plan for wellness? Are you utilizing your special gifts to find a sense of meaning and purpose in life?
- Review Step 2 and focus on the amazing interconnectedness of mind, body, spirit, heredity and the environment (physical and

social). Are you effectively chasing away the "tigers in your path" and the "tigers in your mind"? Are there any "crouching tigers" in your path and mind? Are you doing all you can to keep your life balanced?

- Review Step 3 and take time to reflect on the Mind/Brain-Gut Connection. Is your gut expressing the emotional stress response you are afraid to deal with? Are you using your awareness of triggers/stressors to begin eliminating them from your life? Are there triggers you can avoid but choose not to? Are there triggers you can't avoid but pretend that you can? Are you trying to become more conscious of your feelings so they don't silently wreak havoc on your body?

- Review Step 4 and focus on the Health Mug. Are you aware of the things that are filling up your mug? Are you letting other people dump their "stuff" into your mug? Are you dealing with your unfinished business? Are your lifestyle choices healing or harming you? Are you draining off your unresolved grief or sadness before it causes your mug to overflow? Are your spiritual choices bringing you a greater sense of connection, purpose and meaning in your life?

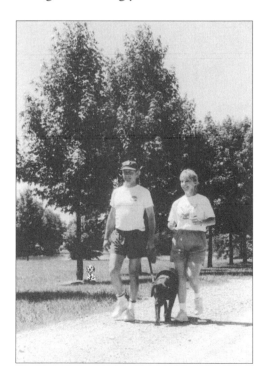

- Review Step 5 and develop a plan for health. Are you exercising regularly? Have you started eating consciously and nutritionally? Are you building your physical strength with a good resistance exercise program? Building strong muscles will help you to feel emotionally and spiritually strong. Are you taking care of the body that houses your soul? Have you reduced your intake of caffeine and alcohol? If you smoke, have you picked a quitting date?

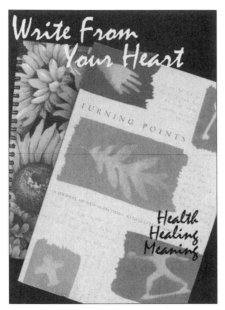

**Never Underestimate the Power of Journaling**

- Review Step 6 and take care of your mind and spirit. Are you keeping a journal yet? Are you spending five minutes at the end of the day reviewing all the things for which you have to be grateful? Are you doing deep breathing exercises and invoking the relaxation response? Are you watching your negative thoughts and eliminating your cognitive distortions? Are you using the ABCDE technique to change your negative attitudes and beliefs into optimistic ones? Are you cultivating positive thoughts, attitudes and beliefs?

Healing is about being your true self—not the part of you covered in mud—but the part of you that shines through like a precious jewel.

The next chapter will introduce you to gastroenterologists, "centers of excellence" and additional resources on IBS and functional gut symptoms and syndromes.

# Chapter 39

## *Gastroenterologists, Centers of Excellence and Resources*

> People handle their fear of change in different ways,
> but the fear is inescapable if we are to change.
> – *The Road Less Traveled*
> M. Scott Peck, M.D.

Most likely, you have been working on your IBS with a family practitioner, internist or pediatrician. This is the best place to start. However, if you are not able to develop a partnership or are not stepping in the direction of symptom relief and healing, then you might want to ask for a referral to a gastroenterology specialist or to a Center of Excellence and review other patient education and support resources.

## How Healing Occurs

Having a good relationship with a primary care doctor is vital. Your primary care doctor is trained to focus on you as a whole person and build a true partnership and collaboration with you and your specialist. Unfortunately, not all physicians have a good understanding of how to help patients with IBS. Your doctor should be interested in you and in trying to help you. If you are not making reasonable progress in a reasonable amount of time, you may need to consider seeing another physician. Some physicians will be better able to provide counseling, support and treatment, including medication. However, it may be necessary for your doctor to refer you to a specialist in the field of digestive medicine—like a gastroenterologist.

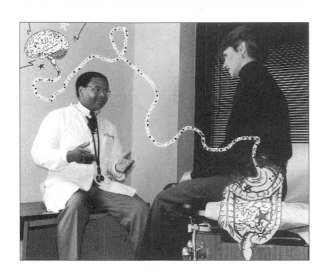

# What Is a Gastroenterologist?

A gastroenterologist is a medical doctor who specializes in the care of people with digestive tract problems. A gastroenterologist first trains as a specialist in internal medicine, which takes at least three years. Then, he or she spends at least two more years learning how to diagnose and treat digestive tract disorders and use high-tech diagnostic and treatment tools such as endoscopes (a flexible tube with a built-in light which permits the doctor to view the inside of the digestive system and perform some surgical procedures through the tube). Learn more about gastroenterologists.

Some gastroenterologists have a special interest in the diagnosis and care of patients with functional gut disorders like IBS. Talk to your doctor and to other people to find the best specialist for you. Always be sure you check with your doctor and insurance carrier to see if any restrictions apply to you.

# Centers of Excellence

Some medical centers specialize in the diagnosis and treatment of IBS and other functional gut syndromes and provide helpful educational information, materials and resources. Two centers of excellence that we recommend:

- **The University of North Carolina Center for Functional GI & Motility Disorders**
  Douglas A. Drossman, M.D. and William E. Whitehead, M.D., Co-Directors
  CB #7080, 778 Burnett-Womack Building
  Chapel Hill, NC 27599-7080
  Phone: (919) 966-0144 • Fax: (919) 966-8929
  Internet: http://www.med.unc.edu/medicine/fgidc/

- **UCLA/CURE Neuroenteric Disease Program**
  Emeran Mayer, M.D., Director
  11301 Wilshire Boulevard
  Building 115, Room 223
  Los Angeles, California 90073
  Phone: (310) 312-9276 • Fax: (310) 794-2864
  Internet: http://www.med.ucla.edu/ndp/

# Resources

There are many patient education and support resources that are available. Here are two excellent resource centers:

- **International Foundation for Functional Gastrointestinal Disorders (IFFGD)**
  Nancy Norton, President and Founder
  IFFGD, P.O. Box 17864
  Milwaukee, WI 53217
  Phone: (888) 964-2001, (414) 964-1799 • Fax: (404) 964-7176
  Internet: http://www.iffgd.org/

- **Irritable Bowel Syndrome (IBS) Self Help Group**
  Jeffrey Roberts, President and Founder
  P.O. Box 94074
  Toronto, Ontario
  CANADA M4N 3R1
  Phone: (416) 932-3311 • Fax: (416) 932-8909
  Internet: http://www.ibsgroup.org/

Learn more about centers of excellence.

Now let's look at other professionals who may help you with your IBS.

# Chapter 40
## *Other MindBodySpirit Professionals*

> Indeed, no leap is possible: not because of an
> unbridgeable gulf between mind and body, but
> because at the archaic level the body is the mind.
> — *Love and Its Place in Nature: A Philosophical
> Interpretation of Freudian Psychoanalysis*
> Jonathan Lear

Caregivers other than physicians may be able to help in the management of your IBS. These caregivers fall into three basic categories: (1) those who work on the *body* at the level of touch (bodyworkers), (2) those who work on the *mind* at the level of talk ("mind" workers) and (3) those who work on the *spirit* at the level of transcendence ("spirit" workers). Including one—or all three—of these professionals in your plan for health can lead to unprecedented improvement.

## Bodyworkers

For centuries, healing has been associated with the use of the hands. Some feel that modern medicine has literally lost "touch" with patients by failing to include manipulation and massage in treatment programs for stress related disorders like IBS. The professionals who reincorporate touch into the healing equation are called bodyworkers. Bodyworkers use touch, manipulation or massage to help you heal.

Bodyworkers include physical therapists, chiropractors, osteopaths, massage therapists, craniosacral therapists, Rolfers, Hellerworkers and practitioners of acupressure, the Alexander technique, Feldenkrais

Method and Therapeutic Touch. For more information on the differences between these techniques, consult the excellent resource book *Alternative Medicine: The Definitive Guide*, by Burton Goldberg.

These practitioners are usually very knowledgeable about how your physical body holds stress at a cellular level. They can help you release body tension of which you may be unaware. Remember that your physical body holds emotions even when your conscious mind does not experience them as feelings. Bodyworkers can help you to find the places in your body that may be "holding" your pain and inhibiting your progress. By releasing this stress, they help free you from the "crouching tigers" in your MindBodySpirit Connection.

Some bodyworkers are traditional in their approach and focus only on your body. Other bodyworkers are more holistic and incorporate emotional release in their physical massage and bodywork. As understanding of the MindBodySpirit Connection grows, these holistic bodyworkers will become a vital asset to any comprehensive program for health and wellness.

As in any field, there are good and bad practitioners. If you decide to use a bodyworker, it is important that you work with one who has appropriate professional education, certification and experience. Skill level varies dramatically from practitioner to practitioner. Don't be afraid to ask about their training, credentials and experience. Also, trust your intuition by choosing a body worker who seems to truly care for you.

# "Mind" Workers

Just as bodyworkers can help relieve your body stress, "mind" workers can help relieve your mental stress. Mostly through talk therapy (although psychiatrists may use medications), they help you uncover disruptive thoughts, unconscious memories and core beliefs that inhibit your healing. The therapeutic benefit of a good "mind" worker cannot be emphasized enough. "Mind" workers include psychologists, psychiatrists, therapists, social workers and counselors.

Many people are afraid to go to a therapist because they feel like it makes them a failure or means that they are weak, wimpy or mentally ill. The truth is, we are all mentally ill in the sense that the stresses of daily life can throw even the strongest and clearest mental attitude out of alignment. Seeing a "mind" worker is like getting a mind/brain neuromatrix alignment. Your mind, body and spirit will steer much more clearly because of it.

# "Spirit" Workers

"Spirit" workers include pastors, priests, ministers, rabbis, chaplains, gurus and mentors who can help you improve the level of your spiritual health. "Spirit" workers help you to find a greater sense of purpose and meaning in life. They help you to identify your unique and special gifts and guide you in using those gifts in a productive and meaningful way. "Spirit" workers practice at the level of transcendence, which means the ability to rise above or go beyond the limits of physical or material existence. Transcendence is about making the invisible qualities of spirit or soul visible in your daily life. Transcendence helps you to find a greater sense of appreciation for the mystery of life, the wonder and awe of simple things. Abraham Joshua Heschel, religious philosopher and scholar, says that a sense of awe allows you to "feel in the rush of the passing, the stillness of the eternal . . . to sense in small things, the beginning of infinite significance." Spiritual growth helps you to transform the invisible qualities of love, kindness, compassion and awe into visible acts of daily life. It is in this transformation that true spiritual health resides.

In the next chapter, you will learn about chronic pain management centers that may be able to help you.

# Chapter 41
## *Chronic Pain Management*

**Don't deny the diagnosis. Try to deny the verdict.**
*– Head First, The Biology of Hope*
Norman Cousins

People who have chronic pain of any type may only be able to "see" the world by what the mind "allows" them to experience. IBS and other chronic pain disorders may require multidisciplinary treatment through specialized treatment centers like chronic pain management programs. This is particularly useful for those with the most complicated psychosocial issues, including matters involving disability.

## The Strain of Pain

The effort to cope with pain leads to stress-related symptoms, fatigue, sleep difficulties and problems with appetite and weight control. Relationships with friends, coworkers and family often suffer. Fear, anxiety, physical tension and depression are common in IBS and can actually increase abdominal pain and discomfort. A vicious cycle begins as your pain leads to psychological distress, which leads back to more pain and increased sensitivity to pain.

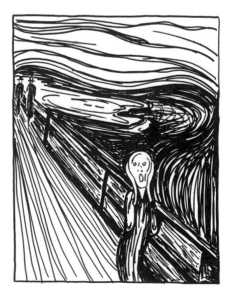

# Chronic Pain Program

A chronic pain program can help you improve the quality of your life, decrease your pain and distress and reduce your visits to the doctor. You can gain a greater sense of mastery over your pain. Many multidisciplinary chronic pain management programs are available throughout the country.

The program that we recommend is the Mind/Body Medical Institute at New England Deaconess Hospital in Boston and Harvard Medical School, under the leadership of Herbert Benson, M.D. The website is www.mbmi.org. The Mind/Body Medical Institute can direct you to an affiliated local institute. Learn more about chronic pain programs.

# Chronic Pain Workbook

If you cannot participate in a pain management program, try reading the book, *Managing Pain Before It Manages You,* by Margaret A. Caudill. This is a pain management program in workbook form. The program is used by patients and health professionals at the New England Deaconess Hospital in Boston, at the Hitchcock Clinic in Nashua, New Hampshire, and at Mind/Body Medical Institute affiliates around the country.

In the next chapter, we'll discuss issues related to determination of disability.

# Chapter 42
## *Disability Determination*

Physicians should encourage . . . patients to
continue to work, since there is evidence in
many chronic pain disorders that disability
adversely affects long term outcome.
– Don L. Goldenberg, M.D.
Professor of Medicine
Tufts University School of Medicine

We strongly advocate that patients with IBS continue to work, especially since studies show that being on disability with IBS and many other chronic pain disorders adversely affects long-term outcome (satisfaction, quality of life and comfort).

## Workers' Compensation

Even though the stress of work may aggravate symptoms, IBS usually occurs independent of a work situation. However, you may choose to pursue compensation under the rules of the Bureau of Workers' Compensation. To receive benefits, you'll need to meet these criteria.

- *A qualified physician must diagnose IBS.* Usually this will be a gastroenterologist with significant experience in the treatment of this disorder.
- *The date of onset of IBS must be established.* Did it occur while the individual was employed or was it a pre-existing condition and present when the individual was hired? There can be considerable dispute as to exactly when the IBS began.

- *The IBS must be associated with a specific work-related event.* Otherwise, it may be difficult to prove that the IBS was actually caused by workplace factors.
- *The degree to which IBS has disabled the individual must be quantified.* It is often difficult to determine and document the amount of physical impairment or disability a person experiences, especially when the physical examination and test results are normal. The physician can use the American Medical Association Guide to Permanent Impairment to quantify the degree of disability. In most cases, it is beneficial to the person making a claim to work with a physician who specializes in IBS.
- *A qualified doctor must provide the prognosis.* The prognosis is the doctor's best estimate—based upon patient information, observation and experienced clinical judgment—of how much ability the individual will be able to recover through proper treatment. The prognosis is a professional opinion based upon estimates of the duration and complexity of the disorder as well as the individual's motivation and compliance with the treatment plan.

## Social Security

Qualifying for Social Security benefits related to IBS may be difficult. As with Workers' Compensation, a person making a Social Security claim should be ready to document the existence of IBS, the date of onset of the disorder, the degree of disability experienced and the prognosis.

However, other factors also come into play with Social Security. Advanced age may compound the effects of pain and discomfort in IBS. Furthermore, education, job training, job experience and the opportunity to pursue alternative work opportunities may figure into the resolution of a Social Security claim.

Individuals whose claims have been filed and rejected may want to seek professional advice from an attorney about appealing the rejection. An appeal guided by an attorney may bring about another case review and ultimately a change in the determination of the original claim.

# Don't Dis-"able" Your MindBodySpirit Connection

When you choose disability, you may be choosing to dis-"able" your MindBodySpirit Connection. This leaves you a helpless victim of a physical disorder—and minimizes the chances that you will ever achieve the level of physical health, emotional peace and spiritual tranquility that attracted you to this book in the first place. If you are unfulfilled at work or overstressed because of a toxic work environment, quit and find another job. But don't quit on yourself. Don't disable yourself. Instead, enable yourself by taking charge of your life and your destiny.

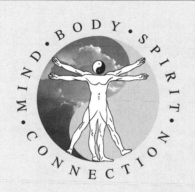

"Much of your pain is self-chosen.
It is the bitter potion by which the physician within you heals your sick self.
Therefore trust the physician, and drink his remedy in silence and tranquillity:
For his hand, though heavy and hard, is guided by the tender hand of the Unseen,
And the cup he brings, though it burn your lips, has been fashioned of the clay which the Potter has moistened with His own sacred tears."
– Kahlil Gibran, *The Prophet*
(New York: Alfred A. Knopf, 1923)

We have one final word—and that word is YOU! This book is about you and what you can do for yourself within the MindBodySpirit model. Knowledge is power and is usually as important as medicine. We believe this book can be our guide by providing you with the information you need to overcome your illness and to be healthier than you have ever been before. You are the healer. It's up to YOU.

# Resources

Benson, Herbert, M.D. *Timeless Healing: The Power and Biology of Belief.* New York: Scribner, 1996.

Bradshaw, John E. *Healing the Shame That Binds You.* Palm Harbor, FL: Health Communications, 1988.

Brody, Howard. *The Placebo Response: How You Can Release the Body's Inner Pharmacy for Better Health.* New York: HarperCollins Publishers, 2000.

Caudill, Margaret A., M.D., Ph.D. *Managing Pain Before It Manages You.* New York: The Guilford Press, 1995.

Cloud, Henry, M.D., and Townsend, John, M.D. *Boundaries: When to Say Yes, When to Say No to Take Control of Your Life.* Grand Rapids, MI: Zondervan Publishing House, 1992.

Cooper, Kenneth. *Aerobics* (out of print).

Cousins, Norman. *Anatomy of an Illness as Perceived by the Patient.* New York: Bantam, 1979.

Cousins, Norman. *Head First: The Biology of Hope.* New York: E.P. Dutton, 1989.

Dacher, Elliott S., M.D. *Intentional Healing.* New York: Marlowe & Company, 1991, 1996.

Dalai Lama, and Cutler, Howard C. *The Art of Happiness.* New York: Riverhead Books, 1998.

Damasio, Antonio R. *Descartes' Error: Emotion, Reason, and the Human Brain.* New York: G.P. Putnam's Sons, 1994.

Damasio, Antonio R. *The Feeling of What Happens: Body and Emotion in the Making of Consciousness.* Orlando: Harcourt, Inc., 1995.

Darden, Ellington, Ph.D. *Body Defining.* Chicago: Contemporary Books, 1996.

Darden, Ellington, Ph.D. *Living Longer Stronger.* New York: The Berkley Publishing Group, 1995.

Dossey, Larry, M.D. *Reinventing Medicine: Beyond Mind-Body to a New Era of Healing.* New York: HarperCollins Publishers, 1999.

Frankl, Viktor E. *Man's Search for Meaning.* Boston: Beacon Press, 1992.

Goldberg, Burton. *Alternative Medicine: The Definitive Guide.* Puyallup, WA: Future Medicine Publishing, 1998.

Goleman, Daniel. *Emotional Intelligence.* New York: Bantam Books, 1997.

Janowitz, Henry D. *Good Food for Bad Stomachs.* New York: Oxford University Press, 1997.

Koenig, Harold G., M.D. *The Healing Power of Faith.* New York: Simon & Schuster, 1999.

Kubler-Ross, Elisabeth, M.D. *On Death and Dying*. New York: Scribner, 1997.

Ledoux, Joseph. *The Emotional Brain: The Mysterious Underpinnings of Emotional Life*. New York: Touchstone Books, 1998.

Levine, Stephen. *Healing Into Life and Death*. New York: Anchor Press, 1989.

Martin, Paul, M.D. *The Healing Mind: The Vital Links Between Brain and Behavior, Immunity and Disease*. New York: St. Martin's Press, 1997.

McGraw, Phillip C., Ph.D. *Life Strategies: Doing What Works, Doing What Matters*. New York: Hyperion Books, 2000.

Moyers, Bill. *Healing and the Mind*. New York: Doubleday, 1979.

Neimark, Neil F., M.D. *The Handbook of Journaling: Tools for the Healing of Mind, Body & Spirit*. Irvine, CA: R.E.P. Technologies, 2000.

Newberg, Andrew, M.D., D'Aquili, Eugene G., Ph.D., and Rause, Vince. *Why God Won't Go Away: Brain Science and the Biology of Belief*. New York: Ballatine Books, 2001.

Pert, Candance B., Ph.D. *Molecules of Emotion: Why You Feel the Way You Feel*. New York: Scribner, 1997.

Reaven, Gerald M., M.D. *Syndrome X: Overcoming the Silent Killer that Can Give You a Heart Attack*. New York: Simon & Schuster, 2000.

Reaven, Gerald M., M.D., and Strom, Terry Kristen, M.B.A., and Fox, Barry, Ph.D. *Syndrome X, The Silent Killer: The New Heart Disease Risk*. New York: Fireside, 2001.

Salt, William B. II, M.D., and Season, Edwin H., M.D. *Fibromyalgia and the MindBodySpirit Connection*. Columbus, OH: Parkview Publishing, 2000.

Sapolsky, Robert M. *Why Zebras Don't Get Ulcers*. New York: W.H. Freeman and Company, 1994, 1998.

Sarno, John E., M.D. *The Mindbody Prescription: Healing the Body, Healing the Pain*. New York: Warner Books, Inc., 1998.

Schneerson, Menachem Mendel. (Adapted by Simon Jacobson.) *Toward a Meaningful Life: The Wisdom of the Rebbe*. New York: William Morrow & Company, 1995.

Seligman, Martin E., Ph.D. *Learned Optimism*. New York: Pocket Books, 1998.

Shorter, Edward. *Doctors and Their Patients: A Social History*. Piscataway, NJ: Transaction Publishing, 1991.

Simonton, Carl O., M.D., Matthews-Simonton, Stephanie, and Creighton, James L. *Getting Well Again*. New York: St. Martin's Press, 1978.

Smith, Huston. *The World's Religions*. San Francisco: Harper San Francisco, 1992.

Thomas, Lewis. *The Lives of a Cell: Notes of a Biology Watcher*. New York: Viking Press, 1974.

Weil, Andrew, M.D. *Natural Health, Natural Medicine*. New York: Houghton Mifflin Company, 1995.

# My Daily Journal

Date: _____

| Type of Symptom | Time | Severity |
|---|---|---|
| | | |

**Symptoms**
Record type of symptom (e.g., diarrhea, constipation, cramping, gas, nausea, anxiety, shakiness, fatigue, headache, etc.), time (e.g., 8 a.m., after dinner, at a meeting, etc.) and severity (on a scale from 1 to 10, with 1 = mild and 10 = severe).

**Mind and Life**
Describe your thoughts, feelings, stresses, memories and what is happening in your life at the time you experience your symptoms.

**Analysis**
Describe any impressions you have about the relationship of your symptoms to your mental outlook and life events.

**Reprogramming Statements**
Write down a positive statement that speaks to your mind, body and spirit. It can be a healing quote you read or a positive statement you created. Reprogramming statements help you transform your negative thoughts into positive, healing ones. (Example: "I acknowledge my power to heal and accept responsibility for my health.")

# Index

# Index

# Index

# Notes

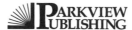

# Discover Parkview Publishing Online!

Finally, a website to put you on the road to recovery . . .

 **www.parkviewpub.com**

Your Online Resource for MindBodySpirit
Connection Symptoms and Syndromes

Created and Edited by Dr. Bill Salt

Log on to the friendly online resource for the latest information and help with:

- Irritable Bowel Syndrome (IBS)
- Other functional gastrointestinal disorders, including
  - Abdominal bloating and distention
  - Abdominal Pain Syndrome (FAPS)
  - Chest pain of presumed esophageal origin
  - Dyspepsia
  - Excessive gas
  - Globus
  - Nausea and vomiting
  - Heartburn
  - Gallbladder and biliary pain
  - Rectal pain
- Bladder and gynecologic symptoms and syndromes
- Fibromyalgia
- Other Functional symptoms and syndromes

All topics found in this book that are indicated by our computer icon
are discussed on our website. You can also find out more about these
Parkview Publishing books on our website:

- *Irritable Bowel Syndrome and the MindBodySpirit Connection*
- *Fibromyalgia and the MindBodySpirit Connection*
- *From IBS to Wellness* (a journal for you to write in)

We invite you to visit, browse and find comfort . . .

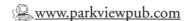 www.parkviewpub.com

283

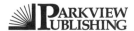

# Parkview Publishing Book Registration

We want to hear from you!

Visit 🖥 www.parkviewpub.com to register this book and tell us how you liked it!

- Sign up to receive a free e-mail copy of our quarterly **Your** Health-**Now! Newsletter**
- Give us feedback about this book – tell us what was most helpful, what was least helpful, or what you'd like to ask the authors and us to change!
- Dr. Salt and Parkview Publishing are deciding on a prioritized list of other MindBodySpirit Syndromes to write about. Let us know what you'd like us to write about next.

Your feedback helps us determine what books to publish, tells us what to add and delete as we revise our books, and lets us know whether we're meeting your needs as a Parkview Publishing reader. You're our most valuable resource, and what you have to say is important to us!

You can also receive a copy of <u>Your</u> HealthNow! Newsletter if you let us know what you think by sending us a letter at the following address:

Parkview Publishing Book Registration
Parkview Publishing
P.O. Box 09784
Columbus, OH 43209-0784

Together We Can Help You Heal